Economics
FOR
Healthcare
Managers

SECOND EDITION

Economics

ᶠᵒʳ Healthcare

Managers

SECOND EDITION

Robert H. Lee

AUPHA

13 12 11 10 09   5 4 3 2 1

Library of Congress Cataloging-in-Publication Data

Lee, Robert H., 1948-
    Economics for healthcare managers / by Robert H. Lee. — 2nd ed.
    p. ; cm.
Includes bibliographical references and index.
ISBN 978-1-56793-314-7 (alk. paper)
  1. Health services administration—Economic aspects. 2. Medical economics. 3. Managerial
    economics. I. Title.
[DNLM: 1. Health Services Administration—economics. 2. Economics, Medical. W 84.1 L4785e
    2009]
    RA427.L44 2009
    362.1068'1—dc22
    2009001332

The paper used in this publication meets the minimum requirements of American National Standard for Information Sciences—Permanence of Paper for Printed Library Materials, ANSI Z39.48-1984. ♾™

Found an error or typo? We want to know! Please email it to HAP1@ache.org, and put "Book Error" in the subject line.

For photocopying and copyright information, please contact Copyright Clearance Center at www.copyright.com or (978) 750-8400.

Project manager: Eduard Avis; Acquisitions editor: Eileen Lynch;
Cover design: Gloria Chantell; Interior layout: Putman Productions, LLC

Health Administration Press
A division of the Foundation
    of the American College of
    Healthcare Executives
One North Franklin Street
Suite 1700
Chicago, IL 60606-3529
(312) 424-2800

Association of University Programs
    in Health Administration
2000 14th Street North
Suite 780
Arlington, VA 22201
(703) 894-0940

CONTENTS

DETAILED CONTENTS

PREFACE TO THE SECOND EDITION

I decided to write a second edition of *Economics for Healthcare Managers* for four reasons. The main reason, of course, was that the world has changed. Economics has begun to engage new issues, and some concerns that seemed paramount in 2000 no longer command the same attention. For example, managed care merited a good deal of discussion in 2000. Today, in contrast, managed care is ubiquitous and familiar. It still merits attention, but our understanding of it has changed. An even more striking change has taken place in our understanding of quality. In 2000 the nation was still trying to absorb the messages of *To Err Is Human* (Institute of Medicine 2000); today, improving the quality of health and healthcare is a core responsibility of healthcare managers.

I also thought that additional topics needed to be covered. One topic was forecasting, which I treated only briefly in the first edition. The second edition devotes an entire chapter to forecasting, as this application of economics is important for managers. Another topic that merited a new chapter was the role of government. Government involvement in health and healthcare is an important issue for managers. In addition, this topic offers instructors an opportunity for lively, topical discussion that should prove to be a welcome addition to many classes.

The second edition remains firmly focused on the economics health-care managers need to understand to be effective, but it updates the references and offers students a glimpse into contemporary research. Although many classic citations remain vital, economists have done a great deal of interesting work during the last decade.

Finally, teaching methods have changed. Case analysis has become increasingly common in economics, and the Internet is becoming an integral part of more and more classes. The second edition reflects these changes.

Every chapter includes one or more case studies and a variety of web-based resources for instructors. Additional learning resources are available to instructors on this book's companion website, hosted by Health Administration Press. These include a test bank, chapter discussion questions and answers, PowerPoint lecture slides, additional reading material, and web links. For access information, e-mail hap1@ache.org.

Reference

Institute of Medicine. 2000. *To Err Is Human: Building a Safer Health System.* Washington, DC: National Academies Press.

WHY HEALTH ECONOMICS?

Learning Objectives

After reading this chapter, students will be able to:

- **describe** the value of economics for managers,
- **identify** major challenges for healthcare managers,
- **find** current national and international information about healthcare outcomes, and
- **distinguish** between positive and normative economics.

Key Concepts

- Economics helps managers focus on key issues.
- Economics helps managers understand goal-oriented decision making.
- Economics helps managers understand strategic decision making.
- Economics gives managers a framework for understanding costs.
- Economics gives managers a framework for understanding market demand.
- Economics gives managers a framework for assessing profitability.
- Healthcare managers must deal effectively with risk and uncertainty.
- Healthcare managers must contend with the management problems that insurance presents.
- Information asymmetries create a number of problems for healthcare managers.
- Not-for-profit organizations create unique problems for managers.
- Rapid change in the healthcare system forces managers to lead their organizations into unfamiliar territory on a routine basis.

1.1 Why Health Economics?

Why should working healthcare managers study economics? This simple question is really two questions. Why is economics valuable for managers? What special challenges do healthcare managers face? These questions motivate this book.

Why is economics valuable for managers? There are six reasons. We will briefly touch on each of them to highlight the themes we will develop in later chapters.

1. Economics helps managers focus on key issues. Economics helps managers wade through the deluge of information they confront and identify the data they need.
2. Economics outlines strategies for realizing goals given the available resources. One of the primary tasks of economics is to explore carefully the implications of rational decision making.
3. Economics gives managers ground rules for strategic decision making. When rivals are not only competing against them but watching what they do, managers must be prepared to think strategically (i.e., be prepared to use the insights of game theory).
4. Economics gives managers a framework for making sense of costs. Managers need to understand costs, as good decisions are unlikely without this understanding.
5. Economics gives managers a framework for thinking about value. The benefits of the goods and services successful organizations provide to customers exceed the costs of producing those goods and services. Good management decisions require an understanding of how customers perceive value.
6. Most important, economics sensitizes managers to fundamental ideas that affect the operations of every organization. Effective management begins with the recognition that consumers are sensitive to price differences, that organizations compete to advance the interests of their stakeholders, and that success comes from providing value to customers.

Do benefits exceed the costs?

1.2 Economics as a Map for Decision Making

Economics provides a map for decision making. Maps do two things. They highlight key features and suppress unimportant features. To drive from Des Moines, Iowa, to Dallas, Texas, you need to know how the major highways connect. You do not want to know the name and location of each street in each town you pass through. Of course, what is important and what is unimportant depend on the task at hand. If you want to drive from Burch Street and Ridgeview Road in Olathe, Kansas, to the Truman homestead in Independence, Missouri, a map that describes only the interstate highway system will be of limited value to you. You need to know which map is the right tool for your situation.

Using a map takes knowledge and skill. You need to know what information you need, or you may choose the wrong map and be swamped in extraneous data or lost without key facts. Having the right map is no guarantee that you can use it, however. You need to practice to be able to use a map quickly and effectively. In the same sense, economics is a map for decision making.

Like a map, economics highlights some issues and suppresses others. For example, economics tells managers to focus on incremental costs, which makes understanding and managing costs much simpler, but economics has little to say about the belief systems that motivate consumer behavior. If you are seeking to make therapeutic regimens easier to adhere to by making them more consistent with consumers' belief systems, economics is not a helpful map. If, on the other hand, you want to decide whether setting up an urgent care clinic is financially feasible, economics helps you focus on how your project will change revenues and costs.

Economics also gives managers a framework for understanding rational decision making. By *rational decision making*, we mean making choices that further one's goals given the resources available. Whether those goals include maximizing profits, securing the health of the indigent, or other objectives, the framework is much the same. It entails looking at benefits and costs to realize the largest net benefit. (We will explore this question further in section 1.5.)

Managers must understand costs and be able to explain costs to others. Confusion about costs is common, so confusion in decision making is also common. Confusion about benefits is even more widespread than confusion about costs. As a result, management decisions in healthcare often leave much to be desired.

Economists typically speak about economics at a theoretical level, using "perfectly competitive markets" (which are, for the most part, mythical social structures) as a model, which makes application of economics difficult for managers competing in real-world markets. Yet, economics offers concrete guidance about pricing, contracting, and other quandaries that managers face. Economics also offers a framework for evaluating the strategic choices managers must make. Many healthcare organizations have rivals, so good decisions must take into account what the competition is doing. Will being the first to enter a market give your organization an advantage, or will it give your rivals a low-cost way of seeing what works and what does not? Will buying primary care practices bring you increased market share or buyer's remorse? Knowing economics will not make these choices easy, but it can give managers a plan for sorting through these issues.

1.3 Special Challenges for Healthcare Managers

What special challenges do healthcare managers face? Five issues face healthcare managers more than other managers:

Sidebar 1.1 Not All Management Decisions Are Good Ones

During the 1980s and 1990s, many hospitals acquired physician practices. Nearly all of those hospitals are losing money on what were once profitable practices. Economics provides two important insights into why these acquisition decisions failed to produce desirable results.

First, most purchases were knee-jerk responses to what competitors were doing, rather than well-thought-out business plans. Enamored by the fact that physicians typically generate large inpatient revenues for each dollar of outpatient revenue they generate, hospitals neglected to ask two key questions: How will buying these practices change the amount of inpatient revenues physicians will bring us? Why are physicians willing to sell? We still do not know the answer to the first question. The answer to the second question is simple—hospitals overpaid. They started buying just as practice valuations began dropping as a result of the growth of managed care and increasing competition for patients.

Second, hospitals ignored incentives. Most hospitals converted compensation based on billings to salaries after they acquired practices, which was a significant mistake. Economics reminds us that incentives matter. For physicians whose earnings depend on billings, the marginal patient—the patient squeezed in at the end of the day, or the patient booked in anticipation that someone will cancel—is highly profitable. For physicians whose earnings depend on salaries, the marginal patient is financially unrewarding. Not surprisingly physicians in independent practice saw 28 percent more patients and performed 16 percent more procedures per patient than those in practices owned by hospitals (Greene et al. 2002). In recent years, hospitals have been returning to incentive-based pay. Productivity has turned around as a result, again confirming economists' emphasis on incentives.

Managers of MultiCare Health System in Tacoma, Washington, concluded that continuing losses at MultiCare Medical Group were not acceptable and took steps to improve its financial performance (Stover, Sauter, and James 2004). They decided to return control of operations to the group's physicians and prepared reports to help the physicians improve their financial performance. During a three-year period, MultiCare Medical Group revised its compensation system and productivity goals and significantly improved its profitability. Managers can effect great change if they are armed with good information and given authority to act.

1. The central roles of risk and uncertainty
2. The complexities created by insurance
3. The perils produced by information asymmetries
4. The problems posed by not-for-profit organizations
5. The rapid and confusing course of technical and institutional change

Let's look at each of these challenges in more depth.

1.3.1 Risk and Uncertainty

Risk and uncertainty are defining features of healthcare markets and health-care organizations. Both the incidence of illness and the effectiveness of medical care should be described in terms of probabilities. For example, the right therapy, provided the right way, usually carries some risk of failure. A proportion of patients will experience harmful side effects, and a proportion of patients will not benefit. As a result, management of costs and quality presents difficult challenges. Has a provider produced bad outcomes because he was unlucky and had to treat an extremely sick panel of patients, or because he encountered a panel of patients for whom standard therapies were ineffective? Did his colleagues let him down? Or was he incompetent, sloppy, or lazy? The reason is not always evident.

1.3.2 Insurance

Because risk and uncertainty are inherent in healthcare, most consumers have medical insurance. As a result, healthcare organizations have to contend with the management problems insurance presents. First, insurance creates confusion about who the customer is. Customers use the products, but insurance plans often pay most of the bill. Moreover, most people with private medical insurance receive coverage through their employer (in large part because the tax system makes this arrangement advantageous). Although economists generally agree that employees ultimately pay for insurance via wage reductions, most employees do not know the costs of their insurance alternatives (and unless they are changing jobs, have limited interest in finding out). As a result of the employer plan default, employees remain unaware of the true costs of care and are not eager to balance cost and value. If insurance is footing the bill, most patients choose the best, most expensive treatment—a choice they might not make if they were paying the full cost of care.

In addition, insurance makes even simple transactions complex. Most transactions involve at least three parties (the patient, the insurer, and the provider), and many involve more. To add to the confusion, most providers deal with a wide array of insurance plans and face blizzards of disparate claim forms and payment systems. Increasing numbers of insurance plans have negotiated individual payment systems and rates, so many healthcare providers look wistfully at industries that simply bill customers to obtain revenues. The complexity of insurance transactions also increases opportunity for error and fraud. In fact, both are fairly common.

Despite this bewildering array of insurance plans, many providers still rely on a select few plans for their revenue (a circumstance most managers seek to avoid). For example, most hospitals receive at least a third of their revenue from Medicare. As a result, changes in Medicare regulations or payment methods can profoundly alter a healthcare organization's prospects.

Overnight, changes to reimbursement terms may transform a market that is profitable for everyone to one in which only the strongest, best-led, best-positioned organizations can survive.

1.3.3 Information Asymmetries

Information asymmetries are common in healthcare markets and create a number of problems. An *information asymmetry* occurs when one party in a transaction has less information than the other party. In this situation, the party with more information has an opportunity to take advantage of the party with less information. Recognizing that he or she is at a disadvantage, the party with less information may become skeptical of the other party's motivation and decline a recommendation that would have been beneficial to him or her. For example, physicians and other healthcare providers usually understand patients' medical options better than patients do. Unaware of their choices, patients may accept recommendations for therapies that are not cost-effective or, recognizing their vulnerability to physicians' self-serving advice, may resist recommendations made in their best interest.

From a manager's perspective, asymmetric information means that providers have a great deal of autonomy in recommending therapies. Because providers' recommendations largely define the operations of insurance plans, hospitals, and group practices, managers need to ensure that providers do not have incentives to use their superior information to their advantage. Conversely, in certain situations, patients have the upper hand and are likely to forecast their healthcare use more accurately than insurers. Patients know whether they want to start a family, whether they seek medical attention whenever they feel ill, or whether they have symptoms that indicate a potential condition. As a result, health plans are vulnerable to *adverse selection*—differential enrollment of high-cost customers.

1.3.4 Not-for-Profit Organizations

Most not-for-profit organizations have worthy goals that their managers take seriously, but these organizations can create problems for healthcare managers as well. For example, not-for-profit organizations usually have multiple stakeholders. Multiple stakeholders mean multiple goals, so organizations become much harder to manage, and managers' performance becomes harder to assess. The potential for managers to put their own needs before their stakeholders' needs exists in all organizations but is more difficult to detect in not-for-profit organizations because they do not have a simple bottom line. In addition, not-for-profit organizations may be harder to run well. They operate amid a web of regulations designed to prevent them from being used as tax avoidance schemes. These regulations make setting up incentive-based compensation systems for managers, employees, and contractors (the most important of whom are physicians)

Sidebar 1.2 Questions about Tax Exemptions

Questions about the tax exempt status of hospitals continue to increase. For example, in 2008 the attorney general of Ohio began an investigation of executive pay, billing practices, and provision of charity care. Over 80 percent of hospitals are not-for-profit organizations that do not have to pay federal income tax, state income tax, or local property tax. Recently, the chairman of the House Ways and Means Committee posed the following question: What is the taxpayer getting in return for the tens of billions of dollars per year in tax subsidy? These tax breaks do not appear to result in significantly higher levels of charity care. A recent study by the Government Accountability Office found that the volume of charity care provided by not-for-profit hospitals was only marginally greater than the volume of charity care provided by for-profit hospitals (U.S. Government Accountability Office 2005).

Hospitals began as refuges for the poor, with clearly charitable missions. But the increasing use of hospitals by paying customers, the resulting expansion of the hospital sector, and higher tax rates necessitated clear standards for tax exemption. In 1956 the Internal Revenue Service published a statement requiring that a tax-exempt hospital "be operated to the extent of its financial ability for those not able to pay for the services rendered." In addition, a tax-exempt hospital could not "refuse to accept patients in need of hospital care who cannot pay for such services," nor was it dispensing charity if it operated "with the expectation of full payment" and incurred bad debt as a result of nonpayment.

Thirteen years later, following the introduction of Medicare and Medicaid, the Internal Revenue Service substituted a broader "community benefit" standard, which expanded the definition of activities eligible for tax exemption. After lying dormant for a number of years, the issue resurfaced in the 1980s when local groups began complaining about hospitals' tax exemptions. In the 1990s, the conversion of not-for-profit hospitals to for-profit status seemed to have little effect on taxes (other than increases in local tax revenues), and concern spread.

At present the issue is not settled. Clearly, though, losing tax-exempt status can have a major impact on a hospital's financial circumstances. This issue is a major concern for any not-for-profit manager. Most economists are skeptical of a subsidy without a clear link to the desired outcome. At a minimum, the manager must be able to explain what taxpayers are receiving in return.

more difficult. Further, when a project is not successful, not-for-profit organizations have greater difficulty putting the resources invested in the failed idea to other uses. For example, the trustees of a not-for-profit organization may have to get approval from a court to sell or repurpose its assets. Because of these special circumstances, managers of not-for-profit organizations can always claim that substandard performance reflects their more complex environment.

1.3.5 Technological and Institutional Change

This fifth challenge makes the others pale in comparison. The healthcare system is in a state of flux. Virtually every part of the healthcare sector is reinventing itself, and no one seems to know where the healthcare system is headed. Leadership is difficult to provide if you don't know where you are going. Because change presents a pervasive test for healthcare managers, we will examine it in greater detail.

1.4 Turmoil in the Healthcare System

Why is the healthcare system of the United States in such turmoil? One explanation is common to the entire developed world: rapid technical change. The pace of medical research and development is breathtaking, and the public's desire for better therapies is manifest. These demands challenge healthcare managers to regularly lead their organizations into unmapped territory. To make matters worse, changes in technology or changes in insurance can quickly affect healthcare markets. In healthcare, as in every other sector of the economy, new technologies can create winners and losers. For example, between 2000 and 2007 Medicare payments to ambulatory surgery centers more than doubled (Medicare Payment Advisory Commission 2008). This represents an opportunity for hospitals, but it also represents a threat. Unaffiliated ambulatory surgery centers and physicians' offices are rapidly expanding competitors. In addition, which ambulatory surgeries can be done profitably depends on insurers' payment decisions. What appears profitable today may not be profitable tomorrow if rates change significantly.

1.4.1 The Pressure to Reduce Costs

The economics of high healthcare costs are far simpler than the politics of high healthcare costs. To reduce costs, managers must reallocate resources from low-productivity uses to high-productivity uses, increase productivity wherever feasible, and reduce prices paid to suppliers and sectors where there is excess supply. They also must recognize that cost cutting is politically difficult. Reallocating resources and increasing productivity will cost some people their jobs. Reducing prices will lower some people's incomes. These steps are difficult for any government to take, and many of those who will be affected (physicians, nurses, and hospital employees) are politically well organized.

The fragmentation of healthcare bills compounds the political problem. Most Americans see only a part of the cost of healthcare. A typical American pays his or her share of healthcare costs through a mixture of direct payments for care; payroll deductions for insurance premiums; lower wages; higher prices for goods and services; and federal, state, and

Sidebar 1.3 **Why Is the Pressure to Reduce Healthcare Costs So Strong?**
The United States spends far more on healthcare than other wealthy industrial countries do but, according to health indicators, fares worse than most of them (Cylus and Anderson 2007). Spending per person is nearly double the spending per person in Germany, Canada, and France (see Table 1.1). Differences this large should be reflected in the outcomes of care.

TABLE 1.1
Spending per Person*

Country	1996	2004
Canada	$2,002	$3,165
France	$1,978	$3,139
Germany	$2,222	$3,005
United Kingdom	$1,304	$2,546
United States	$3,708	$6,102

*Spending figures have been converted into U.S. dollars.
SOURCE: Cylus and Anderson (2007).

As you can see in Table 1.2, of the six countries listed, the United States has the shortest life expectancy at birth. In an analysis of potentially avoidable deaths, Nolte and McKee (2008) noted that the United States had a relatively high rate of potentially avoidable deaths a decade ago and had slower rates of improvement than other wealthy industrialized countries. Greater spending should not produce these results.

TABLE 1.2
Life Expectancy at Birth, 2005

Country	Males	Females
Canada	77.8 years	82.6 years
France	76.7 years	83.8 years
Germany	76.2 years	81.1 years
Japan	76.6 years	85.5 years
United Kingdom	76.9 years	81.1 years
United States	75.2 years	80.4 years

SOURCE: Organisation for Economic Co-operation and Development (2008).

local taxes. Because so much of the payment system is hidden, most Americans cannot track healthcare costs. The exceptions, notably employers who write checks for the entire cost of insurance policies and the trustees of the Medicare system, understand the need to reduce costs. Because so few Americans recognize how much their healthcare system costs, the complex system of public regulations and subsidies will change slowly, at best.

1.5 What Does Economics Study?

What does economics study? Economics analyzes the allocation of scarce resources. Although this answer appears straightforward, several definitions are needed to make this sentence understandable. Resources include anything useful in consumption or production. From the perspective of a manager, resources include the flow of services from supplies or equipment the organization owns and the flow of services from employees, buildings, or other entities the organization hires. A resource is scarce if it has alternative uses, which might include another use within the organization or use by another person or organization. Most issues that managers deal with involve scarce resources, so economics is potentially useful for nearly all of them.

Economics focuses on rational behavior—that is, it focuses on individuals' efforts to best realize their goals, given their resources. Because time and energy spent in collecting and analyzing information are scarce resources (i.e., the time and energy have other uses), complete rationality is irrational. Everyone uses shortcuts and rules to make certain choices, and doing so is rational, even though better decisions are theoretically possible.

Much of economics is positive. *Positive economics* uses objective analysis and evidence to answer questions about individuals, organizations, and societies. Positive economics might describe the state of healthcare, for example, in terms of hospital occupancy rates over a certain period. Positive economics also proposes hypotheses and assesses how consistent the evidence is with them. For example, one might examine whether the evidence supports the conjecture that reductions in direct consumer payments for medical care (measured as a share of spending) have been a major contributing factor in the rapid growth of healthcare spending per person. Although values do not directly enter the realm of positive economics, they do shape the questions economists ask (or do not ask) and how they interpret the evidence.

Normative economics often addresses public policy issues, but not always. The manager of a healthcare organization who can identify additional services or additional features that customers are willing to pay for is

---

Sidebar 1.4 Why Does the United States Spend More on Medical Care than Other Wealthy Countries Spend?

Positive

Positive economics has been used answer this question. Spending on a product equals the amount bought times its price, so analysts break down differences in spending into differences in volumes and differences in prices. Analysis shows us that there is little evidence that Americans use more medical care than other wealthy countries, but there is ample evidence that American prices are substantially higher (Docteur, Suppanz, and Woo 2003). For example, compared to patients in other wealthy countries, American patients typically use 27 percent fewer prescriptions but spend 41 percent more, implying that Americans are buying more expensive pharmaceuticals. Similarly, American patients typically have 36 percent fewer physician visits, yet spend 183 percent more (Cylus and Anderson 2007). The price per visit is much higher in the United States.

Americans also spend far more on hospital care, even though they are less likely to be admitted and usually have a shorter stay if they are admitted. Some of the difference can be attributed to prices, but higher levels of staffing and equipment in American hospitals are also factors. Sorting out how much of the difference in the cost per hospitalization is attributable to price differences and how much is attributable to higher levels of staffing and equipment would be categorized as positive economics. Sorting out whether higher levels of staffing and equipment are worth the extra cost takes us into the realm of normative economics.

Normative

---

demonstrating normative economics. Likewise, the manager who can identify features or services that customers do not value is also demonstrating normative economics.

Normative economics takes two forms. In one, citizens use the tools of economics to answer public policy questions. Usually these questions involve ethical and value judgments (which economics cannot supply) as well as factual judgments (which economics can support or refute). A question like, "Should the Medicare program provide coverage for prescription drugs?" involves balancing benefits and harms. Economic analysis can help assess the facts that underlie the benefits and harms but cannot provide an answer. The second form of normative analysis is the basis for this book's content. This form tells us how to analyze what we *should* do, given the circumstances that we face. In this part of normative analysis, market transactions indicate value. For example, we may believe that a drug is overpriced, but we must treat that price as a part of the environment and react appropriately if no one will sell it for less. Most managers find themselves in such an environment.

To best realize our goals within the constraints we face, economics gives us explicit guidance.

1. First, identify plausible alternatives. Breakthroughs usually occur when someone realizes there is an alternative to the way things have always been done.
2. Second, consider modifying the standard choice (e.g., charging a slightly higher price or using a little more of a nurse practitioner's time).
3. Next, pick the best choice by determining the level at which its *marginal benefit* equals its *marginal cost*. (We will explain these terms shortly.)
4. Finally, examine whether the total benefits of this activity exceed the total cost.

Skilled managers routinely perform this sort of analysis. For example, a profit-seeking organization might conclude that a clinic's profits would be as large as possible if it hired three physicians and two nurse practitioners, but that the clinic's profits would be unacceptably low if it did. Profits would fall even further if it increased or decreased the number of physicians and nurse practitioners, so the profit-seeking organization would choose to close the clinic.

Let's back up and define some terms to make this discussion clearer. *Cost* is the value of a resource in its next best use. For example, the cost of a plot of land for a medical office would be the most another user would pay for it, not what it sold for 20 years ago. The next best use of that land might be for housing, for a park, for a store, or for some other use. Usually the next best use of a resource is someone else's use of it, so a resource's cost is the price we must pay for it. If 30 Lipitor tablets are worth $80 to another consumer, that will be our cost for it. *Benefit* is the value we place on a desired outcome. We describe this value in terms of our willingness to trade one desired outcome for another. Often, but not always, our willingness to pay money for an outcome is a convenient measure of value. A *marginal* or an *incremental* amount is the increased cost we incur from using more of a resource or the increased benefit we realize from a greater outcome. So, if a 16-ounce soda costs 89 cents and a 24-ounce soda costs 99 cents, the incremental cost of the larger size is (99 – 89) ÷ (24 – 16), or 1.25 cents per ounce. A rational consumer might conclude that:

1. the incremental benefit of the larger soda exceeds its incremental cost and buy the larger size;
2. the incremental cost of the larger soda exceeds its incremental benefit and buy the smaller size; or
3. the total benefit of both sizes was less than their total cost and buy neither.

Remember, however, that rational decisions are defined by the goals that underpin them. A consumer with a train to catch might buy an expensive small soda at the station to save time.

1.6 Conclusion

Why should healthcare managers study economics? To be better managers. Economics offers a framework that can simplify and improve management decisions. This framework is valuable to all managers. It is especially valuable to clinicians who assume leadership roles in healthcare organizations.

Managers are routinely overwhelmed with information, yet lack the key facts that they need to make good decisions. Economics offers a map that makes focusing on essential information easier.

Homework

1.1   Why is the idea that value depends on consumers' preferences radical?

1.2   Mechanics usually have better information about how to fix automobiles than their customers. What sorts of problems does this advantage create? Do mechanics or their customers do anything to limit these problems?

1.3   A mandatory health insurance plan costs $4,000. There are three workers. One gets $24,500 in employment income and $500 in investment income. One gets $48,000 in employment income and $2,000 in investment income. The third gets $68,000 in employment income and $7,000 in investment income. A premium-based system would cost each worker $4,000. A wage-tax based system would cost each worker 8.5 percent of wages. An income-tax based system would cost each worker 8 percent of income. For each worker, calculate the cost of the insurance as a share of total income.

	$24,500	$48,000	$68,000
E = Employment income			
I = Investment income	$ 500	$ 2,000	$ 7,000
P = Premium cost of insurance	$ 4,000	$ 4,000	$ 4,000

Premium as a percentage of income = $P/(E + I)$
W = Wage tax cost of insurance = $0.085 \times E$
Wage tax as a percentage of income = $W/(E + I)$
T = Income tax cost of insurance = $0.080 \times (E + I)$
Income tax cost as a percentage of income = $T/(E + I)$

1.4 Which plan would be fairer?

1.5 Which of the preceding questions can you answer using positive economics?

1.6 For which must you use normative economics?

1.7 Below are data for Australia, Canada, and the United States.

    a. How did female life expectancy at birth change between 1995 and 2005?

    b. How did expenditure per person change between 1995 and 2005?

    c. What conclusions do you draw from these data?

    d. If you were the "manager" of the healthcare system in the United States, what would be a sensible response to data like these?

	Life Expectancy			Expenditure per Person		
	1995	*2005*	*Change*	*1995*	*2005*	*Change*
Australia	80.8	83.3		$2,056	$3,080	
Canada	81.1	82.7		$2,543	$3,496	
United States	78.9	80.4		$4,593	$6,498	

Life expectancy is female life expectancy at birth.
Expenditure per person has been translated into US$ and adjusted for inflation.

Chapter Glossary

Cost. The value of a resource in its next best use

Incremental. A small change from the current situation

Marginal. A small change from the current situation

Marginal analysis. Assessment of the effects of small changes in a decision variable (such as price or the volume of output) on outcomes (such as costs, profits, or the probability of recovery)

Marginal cost pricing. The use of information about marginal costs and the price elasticity of demand to set profit-maximizing prices

Marginal or incremental cost. The cost of producing an additional unit of output

Normative economics. Using values to identify the best options

Positive economics. Using objective analysis and evidence to answer questions about individuals, organizations, and societies

Rational decision making. Choosing the course of action that gives you the best outcomes, given the constraints you face

Scarce resources. Anything useful in consumption or production that has alternative uses

References

Cylus, J., and G. F. Anderson. 2007. "Multinational Comparisons of Health Systems Data, 2006." The Commonwealth Fund. [Online information; retrieved 11/14/08.] www.commonwealthfund.org.

Docteur, E., H. Suppanz, and J. Woo. 2003. "The US Health System: An Assessment and Prospective Directions for Reform." [Online information; retrieved 1/28/08.] www.oecdwash.org/PDFILES/us_health_ecowp350.pdf.

Greene, B., J. E. Kralewski, D. N. Gans, and D. I. Klinkel. 2002. "A Comparison of the Performance of Hospital- and Physician-owned Medical Group Practices." *Journal of Ambulatory Care Management* 25 (4): 26–36.

Medicare Payment Advisory Commission. 2008. "Healthcare Spending and the Medicare Program." Medicare Payment Advisory Commission. [Online information; retrieved 11/17/08.] www.medpac.gov/documents/ Jun08DataBook_Entire_report.pdf.

Nolte, E., and C. M. McKee. 2008. "Measuring the Health of Nations: Updating an Earlier Analysis." *Health Affairs* 27 (1): 58–71.

Organisation for Economic Co-operation and Development. 2007. *Health at a Glance 2007: OECD Indicators.* [Online information; retrieved 1/18/08.] puck.sourceoecd.org/vl=6029047/cl=14/nw=1/rpsv/health2007/ g2-1-02.htm.

Stover, S., G. Sauter, and C. James. 2004. "Raising the Performance of Owned Physician Practices." *Healthcare Financial Management* 58 (10): 78–84.

U.S. Government Accountability Office. 2005. "Non-Profit, For-Profit, and Government Hospitals: Uncompensated Care and Other Community Benefits." GAO-05-743T. Washington, DC: U.S. Government Accountability Office.

AN OVERVIEW OF THE
U.S. HEALTHCARE SYSTEM

Learning Objectives

After reading this chapter, students will be able to:

- **articulate** the input and output views of healthcare products,
- **identify** major trends in healthcare,
- **find** current national and international information about healthcare outputs, and
- **apply** marginal analysis to a simple economic problem.

Key Concepts

- Healthcare products are inputs into health and outputs of the healthcare sector.
- The usefulness of healthcare products varies widely.
- Marginal analysis helps managers focus on the right questions.
- Life expectancies have increased sharply in the United States in recent years, but the gains have been smaller and concomitant costs have been higher than in other industrial countries.
- The outputs of the healthcare sector have changed during the last decade.
- Six trends continue to reshape the healthcare sector: (1) overall growth; (2) a shrinking share of direct consumer payments; (3) growth of the number of uninsured; (4) expansion of the outpatient sector; (5) contraction of the inpatient sector; and (6) rapid technological change.

2.1 Input and Output Views of Healthcare

This chapter describes the healthcare system of the United States from an economic point of view and introduces tools of economic analysis. It looks at the healthcare system from two perspectives. The first perspective, called the input view, emphasizes healthcare's contribution to the public's well-being. The second perspective, called the output view, emphasizes the goods and services the healthcare sector produces. In the language of economics, an input is a good or service used in the production of another good or service, and an output is the good or service that emerges from a production process. Products (both goods and services are considered products) are commonly both inputs and outputs. For example, a surgical tool is an input into a surgery and an output of a surgical tool company. Similarly, the surgery itself can be considered an output of the surgical team or an input into the health of the patient.

2.1.1 *The Input View*

The input view of the healthcare system stresses the usefulness of healthcare products. From this perspective, healthcare products are neither good nor bad; they are simply tools used to improve and maintain health. The input view is important because it focuses our attention on alternative ways of achieving our goals, and healthcare products are only one of many inputs into health. Others, such as exercise, diet, and rest, are alternative ways to improve or maintain health. From this perspective, a switch from medical therapies for high blood pressure to meditation or exercise would be based on the following question: Which is the least expensive way to get the result I want? This apparently simple question can be very difficult to answer.

The input view stresses that the usefulness of any resource depends on the problem at hand and other available resources. Whether the health of a particular patient or population will improve as a result of using more healthcare products depends on a number of factors, including the quality and quantity of healthcare products already being used, the quality and quantity of other health inputs, and the general well-being of the patient or population. For example, the effect of a drug on an otherwise healthy 30-year-old is likely to be different from its effect on an 85-year-old who is taking 11 other medications. Or, increasing access to medical care is not likely to be the best way to reduce infant mortality in a population that is malnourished and lacks access to safe drinking water, given the powerful effects of better food and water on health outcomes. Likewise, if the question is, What is the best way to use our resources, given that most preventable mortality is a result of risky behavior?, more medical care is not the answer. All of these examples illustrate that the usefulness of resources varies with the situation.

The economic perspective of *marginal analysis* challenges us to examine the effects of changes on what we do. Marginal analysis proposes questions such as: How much healthier would this patient or population be if we increased use of this resource? How much unhealthier would this patient or population be if we reduced use of this resource? Most management decisions are made on the basis of marginal analysis, although the questions used to arrive at the decisions are often more concrete. For example: What costs would we incur if we increased the chicken pox immunization rate among three-year-olds from 78 to 85 percent, and how much would increased immunization reduce the incidence of chicken pox among preschoolers? Reasonable answers to these questions tell us the cost per case of chicken pox avoided, and we can decide whether we want to use our resources for this proposition. Managers who focus on healthcare products as outputs of their organizations ask the same types of questions, although they frame them differently: How much will profits rise if we increase the number of skilled nursing beds from 12 to 18? What costs would we incur if we added a nurse midwife to the practice, and how would this addition change patient outcomes and revenues? In any setting, marginal analysis helps managers focus on the right questions.

Using estimates from an article on the cost-effectiveness of prevention (Tengs 1996), Figure 2.1 illustrates how variable the effects of medical interventions can be. It estimates how many life years would be saved by spending $1 million on a particular population. (A *life year* is one additional year of life. One person living for nine additional years, and nine persons living for one additional year, equally represent nine life years.) The data indicate that spending $1 million on screening black newborns for sickle cell disease would save more than 4,000 life years but that spending the same amount on screening nonblack, high-risk newborns would save less than ten life years. Figure 2.1 also reminds us that our attitudes toward health are more complex than we sometimes admit. Spending $1 million on mandatory motorcycle helmet laws would save a few more life years than spending $1 million on vaccinating the over-65 population against pneumonia would save, yet the helmet law is controversial and the vaccinations are not. We have to make some choices. Screening nonblack, low-risk newborns for sickle cell disease saves virtually no life years. On rare occasions, though, this screening identifies a non-black, low-risk newborn with sickle cell disease. We cannot avoid a decision about whether the benefits of this intervention are large enough to justify its substantial costs. In different ways, these illustrations remind us that the usefulness of healthcare products varies dramatically.

FIGURE 2.1
How Many Life Years Will $1 Million Save?

Sickle cell screens for black newborns	4,167
Defibrillators in emergency vehicles	2,564
Mandatory motorcycle helmet laws	500
Pneumonia vaccinations for those over age 65	476
Sickle cell screens for nonblack, high-risk newborns	9
Sickle cell screens for nonblack, low-risk newborns	0

SOURCE: These calculations are based on estimates presented in Tengs (1996).

The input view also stresses that changes in technology or prices may affect the mix or amount of healthcare products citizens want to use. For example, lower surgery costs will increase the number of people who choose vision correction surgery rather than eyeglasses. Conversely, advances in pharmaceutical therapy for coronary artery disease might reduce the rate of bypass graft surgeries (and reduce the number of attendant hospital stays).

In the past, healthcare managers did not spent much time on the input view. They were charged with running healthcare organizations well, so products that their organizations did not produce were of little interest. This perception is changing. Our collective rethinking of the role of health insurance makes the input view practical. For example, if offering instruction on meditation reduces healthcare use enough, the chief executive of an insurance plan, the medical director of a capitated healthcare organization, or the benefits manager of a self-insured employer will find it an attractive option. Increasingly, healthcare managers must be prepared to evaluate a wide range of options.

2.1.2 The Output View

New ways of thinking do not always invalidate former perspectives. The output view of the healthcare sector is more relevant than ever. The importance of producing goods and services efficiently has increased. Those struggling with the rising cost of healthcare are increasingly purchasing care from low-cost producers. At present, third parties (i.e., insurers, governments, and employers) have difficulty distinguishing between care that is inexpensive because it is of inferior quality and care that is inexpensive because it is produced efficiently, but their ability to make this distinction is growing. To succeed, managers must lead their organizations to become efficient producers that attract customers. In many organizations, this task will be formidable.

2.2 Health Outcomes

Americans often celebrate their healthcare system as "the best in the world." While parts of the system are superb, the system as a whole needs improvement. As indicated in Chapter 1, the American healthcare system incurs high costs and produces mediocre outcomes. Although the United States spends more on healthcare per person than any other large, developed country, American life expectancy at birth ranks 22nd among the 29 members of a group of industrialized nations called the Organisation for Economic Co-operation and Development (OECD). Only Denmark, the Czech Republic, Mexico, Poland, the Slovak Republic, Hungary, and Turkey trailed the United States

(OECD 2007). (Portugal ranked the same as the United States.) Given the political decision to subsidize healthcare resources for the elderly, female life expectancy at age 65 might represent a fairer test. On this measure, the United States ranked 13th in 2004. Despite this and many other areas of excellence, however, Americans would have difficulty arguing that the United States' healthcare system is the best in the world.

This caustic appraisal should not hide the fact that the health of the American public has improved dramatically. Between 1960 and 2004 the infant mortality rate fell by 74 percent in the United States, and the death rate among new mothers and mothers-to-be fell even more sharply (OECD 2007). Other death rates have fallen as well. Age-adjusted rates of death resulting from cerebrovascular diseases fell by 72 percent, and age-adjusted rates of death resulting from motor vehicle accidents fell by 34 percent. Americans are living longer. Life expectancy at birth rose from 69.7 years in 1960 to 77.8 in 2004, an increase of 7.9 years. (Centers for Disease Control and Prevention 2007.)

From one perspective, this increase in life expectancy reflects impressive performance. From another, it does not compare well to the performance of other industrialized countries. For example, French life expectancy at birth rose from 70.3 in 1960 to 80.3 in 2004. Making the comparison look even less favorable, costs increased more than twice as much in the United States as in France.

This conclusion rests on a simple marginal analysis in which we compare the change in spending to the change in life expectancy. What appears to be higher spending, however, might just be the effects of inflation. To avoid inaccuracies resulting from changes in the value of money, economists use two strategies. The simplest and most reliable strategy reports spending as shares of national income, or *gross domestic product* (GDP). This examination of shares removes the effects of inflation (see Figures 2.2–2.4). When we need to compare dollar amounts, we adjust all the spending figures to a common basis. These inflation-adjusted spending levels are often called *real spending levels*. The price indexes that underlie these adjustments are imperfect, so the adjustments are as well. Consequently, economists are reluctant to make much of small changes in real spending.

To compare French and U.S. spending, we also need to convert figures into a common currency. OECD (2007) regularly publishes estimates of spending per person for a number of countries in U.S. dollars, so we can use these data as a starting point. Converting these figures into inflation-adjusted U.S. dollars, we find that real spending per person in the United States rose from $938 in 1960 to $6,037 in 2004. In contrast, real spending per person in France rose from $440 in 1960 to $3,191 in 2004. Therefore, annual spending in the United States increased by $5,099 per person, and annual spending in France increased by $2,751 per person. This simple marginal

---

Sidebar 2.1 Calculating Inflation-Adjusted Values

Per capita healthcare spending was $7,026 in 2006 and $4,104 in 1997. Did real spending go up? After all, prices generally increased during this period. The Consumer Price Index increased from 152.4 to 201.6, implying that prices rose by 32 percent from 1997 to 2006: 201.6 ÷ 152.4 = 132 percent. To express the 1997 spending figure in inflation-adjusted terms, we multiply it by the value of the Consumer Price Index for 2006 and divide it by the value of the Consumer Price Index in 1997 ($4,104 × 201.6) ÷ 152.4 = $5,429. We conclude that inflation-adjusted spending did go up.

---

analysis does not tell us why costs rose more and life expectancy rose less in the United States, but spending nearly twice as much for a smaller payoff suggests we are not using our resources wisely.

2.3 Outputs of the Healthcare System

In 2006, Americans spent $2.1 trillion on healthcare, meaning that healthcare claimed 16 percent of the nation's output (see Figure 2.2). In 2000, inflation-adjusted healthcare spending totaled $1.4 trillion, or 14 percent of output. Why is how much we spend on healthcare interesting? Is there anything wrong with healthcare spending?

2.3.1 Why Is How Much We Spend on Healthcare Interesting?

How much we spend on healthcare is interesting for two reasons. First, although healthcare is claiming an increasing share of national income

FIGURE 2.2

National Health Expenditures as a Share of Gross Domestic Product

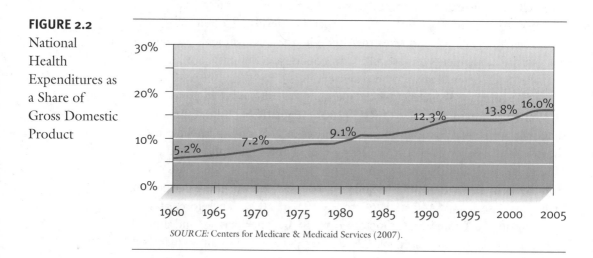

SOURCE: Centers for Medicare & Medicaid Services (2007).

Sidebar 2.2 Comparing Health Outcomes in Utah and Nevada

In 1974, Victor Fuchs compared health outcomes for residents of Utah and Nevada, noting that, despite their many apparent similarities, residents of the two states were at opposite ends of the health spectrum. Residents of Utah were among the healthiest in the nation; residents of Nevada were among the least healthy. Fuchs (1974) argued that the explanation for these health differences "almost surely lies in the different life-styles of the two states."

Despite major changes in the populations of both states, large differentials persist. Focusing on death rates (the crudest but most accurate measures of health), Table 2.1 shows that death rates for adults in Nevada remain much higher. Moreover, the differences are similar to those found by Fuchs.

TABLE 2.1 Excess Death Rates in Nevada over Utah, 1999–2004

	Males	Females
Under 1 year	24%	0%
1–19 years	17%	8%
20–44 years	43%	35%
45–64 years	39%	56%
65–84 years	14%	18%
Over 84 years	–3%	–4%

SOURCE: CDC (2008).

One striking change has taken place: the two states' infant mortality rates have converged. In 1974, Fuchs found infant mortality rates more than 35 percent higher in Nevada, much more than the differential in Table 2.1. This change likely reflects improvements in the treatment of low birth weight (less than 2,500 grams) infants. Differences in infant mortality rates largely depend on the proportion of children with low birth weights, which is heavily influenced by what individuals do, and survival rates among children with low birth weights, which largely reflect effects of the healthcare system (Guyer et al. 1999). The proportion of children with low birth weights is about 21 percent higher in Nevada (Centers for Disease Control and Prevention 2007), so the convergence of infant mortality rates appears to reflect improvements in the treatment of low birth weight infants.

A significant portion of excess mortality in Nevada can be traced to different patterns of alcohol and tobacco use (see Table 2.2). Greater use leads to much larger age-adjusted death rates for malignant neoplasms of the respiratory system (an uncommon disease among nonsmokers) and for chronic liver disease (including cirrhosis).

(continued)

Sidebar 2.2 continued

The consequences of alcohol and tobacco abuse are purely medical issues, but finding ways to reduce the consequences of abuse is a classic problem for those taking the input view of healthcare.

TABLE 2.2

Excess Age-Adjusted Death Rates in Nevada over Utah, 1999–2004

	Males	Females
Malignant neoplasms of the respiratory system	91%	55%
Chronic liver disease and cirrhosis	106%	208%

SOURCE: CDC (2008).

These differences in health outcomes are unlikely to be attributable to differences in healthcare resources. What citizens do (e.g., smoke) and do not do (e.g., exercise) are much more likely to explain these differences. Spending more on healthcare is not the only way to improve outcomes.

worldwide, other industrialized countries appear to be realizing larger health gains while spending less than the United States. Second, the rising share of national income claimed by healthcare has prompted most governments and employers to question whether the benefits of this increased spending warrant it. If not, there is something wrong with healthcare spending. If the benefits of healthcare spending are smaller than the benefits of using our resources in other ways, a shift would be in order. For example, would we be better off if we had spent less on educating new physicians and more on educating new teachers? The *opportunity cost* of producing a product consists of the other goods and services we cannot make instead. The implication is that healthcare need not be bad or worthless for its benefits to be less than its costs, only that it needs to be worth less than some other use of our resources.

Inefficiency is another concern. Seemingly, many healthcare outputs could be produced using fewer resources, and some health outcomes could be realized in ways that use fewer resources. The healthcare system may be wasting resources that have other, more valuable uses.

Case 2.1   **A Pain in the Back**

Americans with back pain are using more painkillers, having more surgeries, and undergoing more imaging studies (magnetic resonance imaging and computed tomography) than ever, yet they do not appear to be feeling better. In 2005, patients with back problems reported more limited functioning than patients did in 1997, even though inflation-adjusted spending was up more than 60 percent (Martin et al. 2008).

Neck and back pain are common, and a majority of adults have an episode during the course of a year. Neck and back pain are also common reasons for physician visits. During these visits, physicians usually (or should) reassure patients that most low back pain improves with conservative treatment (a combination of ice and nonprescription pain relievers, followed by moderate strengthening and stretching exercises that can be done at home without special equipment). Diagnostic imaging is being prescribed more frequently for patients with back and neck pain, even though the value of imaging appears to be limited (Carragee 2005). Few imaging studies yield a definitive diagnosis or a new treatment plan. Furthermore, Medicare data show that rates of back surgery have increased dramatically, even though there is little scientific evidence that surgery is superior to conservative treatment. The United States has the highest rates of back surgery in the world, even though back problems are no more common here than in other countries. In addition, surgery rates also vary greatly between cities. For example, during the 1990s, the back surgery rate for residents of Fort Myers, Florida, was 142 percent higher than the rate for residents of Miami (Weinstein et al. 2004).

Discussion questions:

- If imaging followed by surgery is as effective as conservative therapy, what's wrong with letting physicians and patients do what they want?
- What explains this rise of imaging and surgery for back pain?
- Should insurers take action to reduce surgery rates? Should individuals? Who makes decisions about surgery?
- How do providers' revenues change if imaging and surgery rates rise? How do patients' costs change if imaging and surgery rates rise?
- How do current incentive systems affect physicians' and patients' decisions?

2.3.2 The Shifting Pattern of Healthcare Spending

The mix of healthcare outputs has changed. New technologies and new insurance arrangements are altering what the public buys. Figure 2.3 gives an overview of these shifts.

Hospitals' share of healthcare outputs has been falling since the early 1980s. Even though they have expanded into nontraditional markets and are earning more revenue, hospitals produced slightly less than a third of the output of the healthcare sector in 2006 (Centers for Medicare & Medicaid

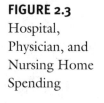

FIGURE 2.3

Hospital,
Physician, and
Nursing Home
Spending

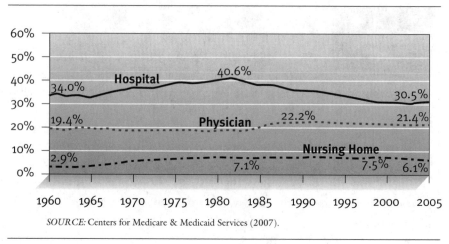

SOURCE: Centers for Medicare & Medicaid Services (2007).

Services 2007). The number of inpatient days has been falling, however, and other healthcare sectors have been expanding rapidly.

Physicians' output share has risen only a little since 1960. This is attributable to the rapid growth in other healthcare sectors, not slowing spending on physicians' services. Inflation-adjusted spending on physicians' services increased by 32 percent between 2000 and 2006 (Centers for Medicare & Medicaid Services 2007). For several reasons, dentists' output share has steadily fallen since 1960. One reason is that cavity control is one of the great healthcare success stories of the last 50 years. The introduction of fluoride toothpaste, fluoridated drinking water, and topical fluoride treatments has significantly reduced the prevalence of tooth decay. In addition, the growth of dental insurance has been slower than the growth of other types of insurance. In 2006, consumers directly paid for 47 percent of dental care. In contrast, consumers paid for only 10 percent of physicians' services.

High drug prices and the implementation of Medicare Part D in 2006 have had significant effects on spending. Furthermore, in the last few years, prescription drug coverage has been paying an increasing amount of the cost of prescriptions. In 1990, consumers directly paid 56 percent of the cost of prescription drugs. In 2006, consumers directly paid for 10 percent of the cost. Yet, as Figure 2.4 shows, spending on prescription drugs claims about the same share of GDP as it did in 1960, and the rate of increase in prices has actually gone down in recent years (Centers for Medicare & Medicaid Services 2007). Most of the growth in spending reflects increased use of pharmaceuticals, not higher prices. There are several reasons for this seeming disconnect. First, consumers are using more inexpensive generic drugs. In 2006, generics represented 63 percent of all prescriptions (Generic Pharmaceutical Association 2008). Second, the prices of many generics have been driven down by intense competition

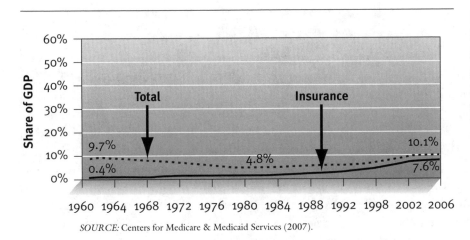

FIGURE 2.4

Pharmaceutical Spending as a Share of National Health Spending

among retailers (e.g., Wal-Mart and Target). Third, pharmaceutical manufacturers have huge start-up costs and low costs per additional dose, so the price per dose is negotiable. Consumers usually pay list price, but insurers generally do not. So, as insurance coverage spreads, the share of discounted transactions increases.

The output of nursing homes has increased more slowly than overall healthcare spending, even though the elderly population has continued to grow. Other options, such as assisted living and home health care, have expanded rapidly.

2.4 Trends Reshaping the Healthcare System

Six trends continue to reshape the healthcare system of the United States. Most of these trends are well known, yet some are so gradual and so much a part of day-to-day operations that even skilled managers tend to ignore them. The trends are:

1. growth of the healthcare sector;
2. shrinking share of direct consumer payments;
3. growth of the uninsured;
4. expansion of the outpatient sector;
5. contraction of the inpatient sector; and
6. rapid technological change.

2.4.1 Growth of the Healthcare Sector

The growth of the healthcare sector has been a feature of American life for most of this century, and it has not stopped. As Figure 2.2 shows, healthcare

Sidebar 2.3 Prescription Drugs and the Consumer Price Index

The Consumer Price Index may overstate the rate of growth of prescription prices. The Bureau of Labor Statistics (2008a), which compiles the Consumer Price Index for prescription drugs, samples 300 retail outlets that are representative of the locations where Americans buy prescription drugs. The outlets include chain pharmacies, neighborhood pharmacies, discount stores, and mail-order firms. The Bureau tracks the prices of 20 representative drugs but faces four major problems in the rapidly changing pharmaceutical market: shifts in insurance coverage, the emergence of generics, the conversion from prescription to over-the-counter status, and the introduction of new drugs. These ongoing changes make constructing a good index of prices more difficult. For example, what should happen to the price index if the price of a branded drug remains $100 but a third of consumers switch to a generic version costing $40? Or, what should happen to the price index if a third of consumers switch to a new drug that costs $120? Presumably this new drug represents a better value than the older, less expensive drug, and the index should reflect this difference. The Bureau has implemented changes to address these issues but is having difficulty keeping up with shifts in the pharmaceutical market.

spending in 1960 claimed only 5.2 percent of national income. In 2006, healthcare spending claimed 16 percent of national income. This continuing expansion has meant two things. One is that a smaller proportion of national income has been available for other purposes. This reduced share is a problem only if consumers feel that the benefits of this added spending are smaller than the benefits of spending the money in some other way. The second implication is that a disproportionate number of new healthcare jobs have been created.

For a typical student, the question of whether this rapid healthcare job growth will continue is more salient than musings about the benefits of added healthcare spending. There are two reasons why the rate of healthcare job creation might slow. First, the expansion of the healthcare sector has slowed somewhat in recent years. Whether this deceleration is a trend remains to be seen, but slower expansion would mean slower job growth. Second, changes in the financing system have increased incentives for the healthcare sector to become more efficient. The simplest way to become more efficient is to use hospital care (which is expensive and labor intensive) only when necessary. This trend is already evident and seems likely to continue. Between 2000 and 2006, jobs in the hospital sector grew about half as fast as other healthcare jobs (U.S. Department of Health and Human Services 2007, Table 105).

Case 2.2

Opportunities in Long-Term Care

Between 2010 and 2050, the number of Americans over age 84 is projected to more than triple (U.S. Census Bureau 2004). As they become more disabled, most elderly people prefer not to move to a nursing home and instead take advantage of other services.

This desire for aging in place is likely to result in rapid growth in several healthcare sectors. One is home health, in which workers provide a wide range of services in clients' homes. Another sector, residential care facilities, is more diverse. For example, continuing care retirement communities have a range of accommodations designed to meet the health and housing needs of residents as these needs change over time. Residents typically sign a long-term contract that provides for housing and nursing care, usually all in one location, enabling seniors to remain in a familiar setting as they grow older. These communities usually include homes for independent living (and contracts with home health agencies to support residents in these homes), assisted living facilities for residents who can no longer live independently, and nursing facilities for residents who require high levels of care.

Even before the start of the demographic tsunami, significant growth had taken place. Between 1998 and 2004, beds in residential care facilities increased by more than 50 percent (Mollica, Johnson-Lamarche, and O'Keeffe 2005), and the number of home health aides and personal care aides increased by 72 percent (Bureau of Labor Statistics 2008b).

One thing is certain. Residential care for the elderly will look different in 20 years. It will claim a much larger share of healthcare spending. It will increasingly focus on the services that residents want. It will face significant labor shortages. And it will be profoundly affected by changes in technology, including devices that assist residents and monitor their safety.

In short, residential care for the elderly will be a sector marked by growth and innovation. As such, it will create multiple opportunities for healthcare managers. These firms require skilled leadership in marketing, facilities management, human resources, clinical care, and many other areas.

Discussion questions:
- Why should a manager stay abreast of major trends like the growth of residential care for the elderly?
- Why might residential care managers not understand what their customers want?
- Why would their lack of understanding matter?
- What could a manager do to better understand what customers want?
- Are there parts of the healthcare sector that will experience slower growth than residential care for the elderly?
- How would a career in a slow-growing sector differ from a career in a fast-growing sector?

2.4.2 Shrinking Share of Direct Consumer Payments

The most consistent force underpinning the evolution of America's health-care system has been the shrinking share of services that consumers pay for directly. As Figure 2.5 shows, consumers directly paid for 49 percent of healthcare bills in 1960 but only 12 percent in 2006. Events that occurred between 1960 and 1975 contributed to this reduction. In 1966, Medicare was introduced and state medical assistance programs were converted to Medicaid. The expansion of private insurance was also a contributing factor. Expanding access to healthcare by reducing direct consumer payments was the goal of policy during this period.

Since 1975, emphasis has been placed on cost control efforts and the increasing number of Americans without health insurance coverage. Yet broader coverage (e.g., expanded pharmacy benefits) has caused the share of spending financed by public and private insurance to steadily increase. Ultimately, consumers pay all healthcare bills. Increasingly, though, they are doing so indirectly via taxes and premiums.

The State Children's Health Insurance Program (SCHIP), which started in 1998, represented the first major expansion of government-funded insurance since 1972. Designed to provide coverage to children in families with incomes too high to be eligible for Medicaid, it also entailed changes in Medicaid designed to increase enrollment. In 1998, spending on these two programs totaled $346 million. In 2006, it totaled $8.4 billion, which is only 0.4 percent of national health expenditures (Centers for Medicare & Medicaid Services 2007).

Medicare Part D, which started in 2006, expanded government-funded insurance much more. Providing prescription drug coverage for Medicare ben-

FIGURE 2.5

Out-of-Pocket, Insurance, and Government Shares of Healthcare Spending

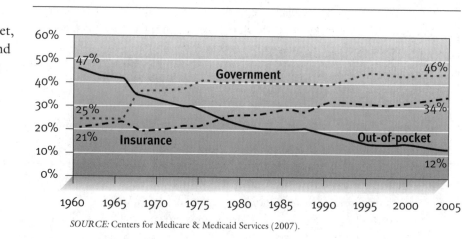

SOURCE: Centers for Medicare & Medicaid Services (2007).

eficiaries, Part D replaced Medicaid coverage for many Medicare beneficiaries. As a result, Medicare spending rose from 17.1 percent of national health expenditures in 2005 to 19.1 percent in 2006 (Centers for Medicare & Medicaid Services 2007). In addition, for the first time in the history of the program, Medicaid spending fell, to 15.8 percent of national health expenditures in 2005 and 14.7 percent in 2006 (a drop of $2.8 billion).

2.4.3 Growth of the Uninsured

Increasing numbers of Americans lack health insurance. In 1984, 30 million residents of the United States under age 65 had no health insurance. By 2006, this number had risen to 47 million, representing 15.8 percent of the population under age 65 (U.S. Census Bureau 2007, Table HIA-2). The number of uninsured would have risen even faster if enrollment in Medicaid and SCHIP had not risen by about 24 million.

The increase in the number of uninsured Americans affects almost all healthcare organizations. Seriously ill, uninsured patients are unlikely to be able to pay their bills. A small number of providers, such as free clinics, public health clinics, public hospitals, and university hospitals, have traditionally served the majority of the uninsured. If the number of uninsured continues to increase, these traditional charity providers could go bankrupt. As a result, these patients may be left with no access to care, or other providers may face significant demands for charity care.

Most of the uninsured population maintains that insurance costs too much. For some, health insurance is worth less than other products. For someone with a low income, good health, few assets, and access to emergency care, insurance is unlikely to be a high priority. He or she will not be willing to pay more than a small sum for coverage. In contrast, someone in poor health with a moderate income will be willing to pay substantially more for insurance, but it may be prohibitively expensive, especially if he or she is not a member of a large group that purchases insurance collectively.

In 2006, over 87 percent of Americans with private insurance were covered through their employers (U.S. Census Bureau 2007, Table H1A-2). Three main reasons account for this statistic. First, U.S. tax laws exclude employer-paid health insurance premiums from taxable income, which nearly halves the after-tax cost of insurance. Second, employment-based insurance sharply reduces insurers' marketing costs. In particular, employment-based insurance allows insurers to spend less to protect themselves against *adverse selection*, which occurs when those who expect high healthcare bills are much more willing to pay for coverage than those who expect low healthcare bills. Third, Americans have repeatedly rejected the idea of health insurance systems run or sponsored by the government.

2.4.4 Expansion of the Outpatient Sector

More and more, complex care is being provided on an outpatient basis by hospital outpatient departments, freestanding facilities, and physicians' offices. Imaging, testing, and many surgeries are no longer inpatient procedures. For example, only 20 percent of surgeries were performed on an inpatient basis in 2005 (American Hospital Association 2006). In 1980, in contrast, inpatient surgeries accounted for 84 percent of the total. Changes in surgical, anesthesia, imaging, and testing technology have driven this change.

2.4.5 Contraction of the Inpatient Sector

Contraction of the inpatient hospital sector is an important trend that is easy to overlook. Figure 2.6 shows that days of care per 1,000 persons have fallen by over 50 percent since 1980, although this contraction has slowed in recent years. Areas with high levels of managed care have much lower rates of hospital use than average, and insurers and health systems are beginning to develop strategies for reducing hospital use still further. Innovations in pharmaceuticals, surgery, and imaging also promise to contribute to sector contraction.

Many healthcare managers are maintaining an inpatient focus. They seek improved hospital operations (a worthy aim) for the purpose of increasing the census (an unlikely result). In most areas, the census of well-managed hospitals will drop more slowly than the census of hospitals that are less well managed. Similarly, in hopes of building the inpatient census, many managers want to start satellite clinics or acquire physician practices. Once the hospital has assumed management of these additions, however, they may not be profitable. The continuing drop in inpatient services will overwhelm the modest increase in referrals that ensues.

FIGURE 2.6

Days of Care per 1,000 People

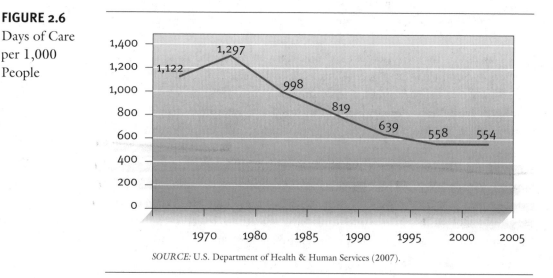

SOURCE: U.S. Department of Health & Human Services (2007).

| Case 2.3 | **Gall Bladder Surgery** |

Changes in imaging and surgical technology allow a surgeon to remove a diseased gall bladder through a few small incisions rather than one long cut through the skin and muscles. In laparoscopic surgeries, the surgeon inserts a lighted scope attached to a video camera (laparoscope) into one of the small incisions to see inside a patient's abdomen. Laparoscopic surgeries usually reduce blood loss, pain, recovery time, and the risk of infection. In addition, patients recover quickly from new, short-acting anesthetics and may be able to go home a few hours after the procedure (Altman 2006).

These changes in technology reduce equipment and personnel costs. They also allow many surgeries to be performed in offices or outpatient surgery centers, which have lower overhead costs (costs not directly related to the procedure). As a result, the cost per surgery is usually lower in an outpatient setting. Insurers typically pay less for outpatient surgery, so they prefer it as much as patients do. Physicians also earn more when they perform a surgery in a facility they partly own.

Despite its widespread appeal, this trend does pose problems. Hospitals are losing market share. In addition, the shift concerns policymakers for three reasons. The first is that, even though the cost per surgery goes down, the number of surgeries increases by more than enough to drive up total expenditure. The added convenience of outpatient surgery appears to have increased the number of patients who are willing to have surgery, and ownership of surgical facilities appears to have affected surgeons' recommendations to patients. The second concern is that the rush to outpatient care adds to the problems of the safety net. Much of the safety net rests on the premise that hospitals will spend some of their profits from inpatient services on care for the uninsured and underinsured. The expansion of the outpatient sector puts this system at risk. The safety net is an odd arrangement from an economic point of view, but dismantling it with no replacement will put vulnerable individuals at greater risk. Finally, there is limited evidence that outpatient surgery is high-quality care. Carefully designed studies have failed to detect differences in the quality of inpatient and outpatient procedures (Johansson et al. 2006), but concerns remain.

Discussion questions:
- Why might patients prefer laparoscopic surgery to traditional surgery?
- Why might surgeons prefer laparoscopic surgery?
- Why is losing market share a problem for a manager?
- What happens to hospital revenues if surgery shifts to outpatient settings?
- Why don't costs go down enough to offset this reduction?
- What options should a hospital manager consider if some surgeons want to invest in an outpatient surgery center?
- Why is paying extra for inpatient care for insured patients an odd way of financing the safety net?

2.4.6 Rapid Technological Change

Rapid technological change is pervasive in healthcare. Only luck will rescue management decisions that ignore it.

Like every sector of society, healthcare struggles to take advantage of the information revolution and demonstrates the paradox of technological change. The essence of the information revolution is that the cost of performing a single calculation has dropped precipitously. As a result, many more calculations are possible, and spending on some types of information processing has increased sharply (e.g., computer games) as spending on other types of information processing has plummeted (e.g., inventory management). Technological advances almost always make a process less expensive, yet spending may rise because volume increases dramatically.

The challenges of the information revolution are even greater in healthcare than in most sectors. Much of the output of the healthcare sector involves information processing, yet relatively few healthcare workers are highly skilled users of computerized information. In addition, healthcare organizations have lagged behind other service organizations in investing in computer hardware, software, and personnel.

The rapid pace of change in other areas further intensifies these already heightened challenges. Healthcare's diagnostic and therapeutic outputs are changing even faster than the organizational structure of the sector, which itself is changing rapidly. In some areas (most notably imaging and laboratory services), technological change is tightly linked to the information processing revolution. In other areas, the links are much looser. For example, advances in information processing speed the development and assessment of new drugs, yet because pharmaceutical innovations can be extremely profitable, powerful incentive for pharmaceutical innovation exists regardless of these advances.

2.5 Conclusion

At some point during the 1980s, a consensus emerged that the United States' healthcare system needed to be redirected despite its many triumphs. Underlying this consensus was the recognition that costs were the highest in the world even though outcomes were not the best in the world.

How the healthcare system should change is much less clear. Managing under such circumstances is stressful, but an awareness of the trends we presented in this chapter should guide any organization's managers, and a number of strategies (such as striving to be the low-cost producer) make sense in almost any environment. These low-risk strategies, and ways to deal with risk and uncertainty, will be discussed in the next chapters.

Homework

2.1   Identify a product that is one organization's output and another organization's input.

2.2   Can you think of any initiatives that reflect the input view of healthcare?

2.3   What's wrong with spending 16 percent of GDP on healthcare?

2.4   Americans spend more on computers than the citizens of other countries, yet this type of spending is seldom described as a problem. Why is spending more on healthcare different?

2.5   U.S. national health expenditure was $7,026 per person in 2006 and $4,790 in 2000. The Consumer Price Index had a value of 201.6 in 2006 and a value of 172.2 in 2000. Adjusted for inflation, how much was spending in 2000?

2.6   U.S. national health expenditure was $148 per person in 1960 and $4,790 in 2000. The Consumer Price Index had a value of 29.6 in 1960 and a value of 172.2 in 2000. In 1960 dollars, how much was spending in 2000?

2.7   How did the state and local government share of national health expenditures change between 2000 and last year? What accounts for this change? Go to www.cms.hhs.gov/NationalHealth ExpendData/02_NationalHealthAccountsHistorical.asp to get data.

2.8   When was the last year that gross domestic product grew faster than national health expenditure? Go to www.cms.hhs.gov/NationalHealth ExpendData/02_NationalHealthAccountsHistorical.asp to get data.

2.9   Your accountants tell you that it costs $400 to set up an immunization program at a preschool and immunize one child against polio. It will cost $460 more to immunize 20 more children. What is the cost per child for the first child? What is the cost per child for these additional 20 children? What is the average cost per child? What concepts do these calculations illustrate?

2.10 A new treatment of cystic fibrosis costs $2 million. The life expectancy of 1,000 patients who were randomly assigned to the new treatment increased by 3.2 years. What is the cost per life year of the new treatment?

2.11 Setting up nurse practitioner clinics to serve 20,000 newborns in Georgia would cost $6 million. This would increase life expectancy at birth from 75.1 to 75.3. How many life years would be gained? What is the cost per life year? Should this program be started?

2.12 Why has the share of healthcare output produced by hospitals fallen? Will this trend continue? What implications does this have for the careers of healthcare managers?

Chapter Glossary

Adverse selection. The willingness of high-risk consumers to pay more for insurance than low-risk consumers (Organizations that have difficulty distinguishing high-risk from low-risk consumers are unlikely to be profitable.)

Input. A good or service used in the production of another good or service

Life year. One additional year of life (A life year can also represent 1/nth of a year of life for n people.)

Managed care. A loosely defined term that includes PPO and HMO plans, sometimes used to describe the techniques insurance companies use

Marginal analysis. Assessment of the effects of small changes in a decision variable (such as price or volume of output) on outcomes (such as costs, profits, or probability of recovery)

Output. A good or service that emerges from a production process

References

Altman, L. K. 2006. "So Many Advances in Medicine, So Many Yet to Come." *New York Times,* December 26.

American Hospital Association. 2006. "The Migration of Care to Non-Hospital Settings: Have Regulatory Structures Kept Pace with Changes in Care Delivery?" [Online information; retrieved 1/25/08.] www.aha.org/aha/trendwatch/2006/twjuly2006migration.pdf.

Bureau of Labor Statistics. 2008a. "Consumer Price Indexes." [Online information; retrieved 2/5/08.] www.bls.gov/cpi/.

———. 2008b. "Occupational Employment Statistics." [Online information; retrieved 1/31/08.] www.bls.gov/oes/oes_dl.htm.

Carragee, E. J. 2005. "Persistent Low Back Pain." *New England Journal of Medicine* 352: 1891–98.

Centers for Disease Control and Prevention. 2007. "Health, United States, 2007." [Online information; retrieved 2/5/08.] www.cdc.gov/nchs/hus.htm.

Centers for Medicare & Medicaid Services. 2007. "National Health Expenditures." [Online information; retrieved 1/24/08.] www.cms.hhs.gov/NationalHealthExpendData.

Fuchs, V. R. 1974. *Who Shall Live? Health, Economics, and Social Choice.* New York: Basic.

Generic Pharmaceutical Association. 2008. "Statistics." [Online information; retrieved 2/5/08.] www.gphaonline.org/Content/NavigationMenu/AboutGenerics/Statistics/default.htm.

Guyer, B., D. L. Hoyert, J. A. Martin, S. J. Ventura, M. F. MacDorman, and D. M. Strobino. 1999. "Annual Summary of Vital Statistics—1998." *Pediatrics* 104 (6): 1229–46.

Johansson, M., A. Thune, L. Nelvin, and L. Lundell. 2006. "Randomized Clinical Trial of Day-Care Versus Overnight-Stay Laparoscopic Cholecystectomy." *British Journal of Surgery* 93 (5): 639–40.

Martin, B. I., R. A. Deyo, S. K. Mirza, J. A Turner, B. A. Comstock, W. Hollingworth, and S. D. Sullivan. 2008. "Expenditures and Health Status Among Adults with Back and Neck Problems." *Journal of the American Medical Association* 299 (6): 656–64.

Mollica, R., H. Johnson-Lamarche, and J. O'Keeffe. 2005. "State Residential Care and Assisted Living Policy: 2004." [Online information; retrieved 1/31/08.] http://aspe.hhs.gov/daltcp/Reports/04alcom.htm#acknow.

Organisation for Economic Co-operation and Development (OECD). 2007. "OECD Health Data 2007—Frequently Requested Data." [Online information; retrieved 2/5/08.] www.oecd.org/document/16/0,3343, en_2649_34631_2085200_1_1_1_1,00.html.

Tengs, T. O. 1996. "Enormous Variation in the Cost-Effectiveness of Prevention: Implications for Public Policy." *Current Issues in Public Health* 2: 13–17.

U.S. Census Bureau. 2004. "U.S. Interim Projections by Age, Sex, Race, and Hispanic Origin." [Online information; retrieved 1/31/08.] www.census.gov/ ipc/www/usinterimproj.

———. 2007. "Health Insurance Coverage Status and Type of Coverage—All Persons by Age and Sex: 1999 to 2006." [Online information; retrieved 1/24/08.] www.census.gov/hhes/www/hlthins/historic/index.html.

U.S. Department of Health and Human Services. 2007. *Health, United States, 2007.* [Online information; retrieved 1/29/08.] www.cdc.gov/nchs/data/hus/ hus07.pdf#summary.

Weinstein, J. N., K. K. Bronner, T. S. Morgan, and J. E. Wennberg. 2004. "Trends and Geographic Variations in Major Surgery for Degenerative Diseases of the Hip, Knee, and Spine." [Online information; retrieved 3/11/08.] www.healthaffairs.org.

AN OVERVIEW OF THE HEALTHCARE FINANCING SYSTEM

Learning Objectives

After reading this chapter, students will be able to:

- **use** standard health insurance terminology,
- **identify** major trends in health insurance,
- **describe** why health insurance is common,
- **describe** the major problems faced by the current insurance system, and
- **find** current information about health insurance.

Key Concepts

- Consumers pay for most medical care indirectly, through taxes and insurance premiums.
- Direct payments for healthcare are often called *out-of-pocket* payments.
- Insurance pools the risks of high healthcare costs.
- Moral hazard and adverse selection complicate risk pooling.
- About 85 percent of the population has medical insurance.
- Most consumers obtain coverage through an employer-sponsored or government-sponsored plan.
- Receiving insurance as a benefit of employment has significant tax benefits.
- Managed care has largely replaced traditional insurance.
- Managed care plans differ widely.

3.1 Introduction

3.1.1 Paying for Medical Care

Consumers pay for most medical care indirectly, through taxes and insurance premiums. Healthcare managers must understand the structure of private and social insurance programs because much of their organizations' revenues will be shaped by these programs. Managers must also be aware that consumers ultimately pay for healthcare products, a key fact obscured by the complex structure of the U.S. healthcare financing system. A prudent manager will anticipate a reaction when healthcare spending invokes higher premiums or taxes, thereby forcing consumers to spend less on other goods and services. Some consumers may drop coverage, some employers may reduce benefits, and some plans may reduce payments. This reaction need not occur if a consensus has emerged in support of increased spending, but even then managers should be wary of the profound effects that changes to insurance plans can mean for them. Finally, managers must consider more than the amount subsidized by insurance. Even though the bulk of healthcare firms' revenues comes from payments for products covered by insurance plans, consumers do pay directly for some products. Consumers directly spent more than $257 billion on healthcare products in 2006. No firm should ignore this huge market.

3.1.2 Indirect Spending

Despite its size, direct consumer spending accounts for only a fraction of total healthcare spending. Figure 3.1 depicts a healthcare market in general terms—consumers directly pay the full cost of some services and part of the costs of other services. These direct payments are often called *out-of-pocket payments*. For example, a consumer's payment for the full cost of a pharmaceutical product, her 20 percent coinsurance payment to her dentist, and her $8 copayment to her son's pediatrician are all considered out-of-pocket payments. Insurance beneficiaries make some out-of-pocket payments for services that are not covered, for services in excess of their policy's coverage limits, or for *deductibles* (amounts consumers are required to spend before their plan pays anything). Another name for out-of-pocket payments is *cost sharing*. Economics teaches us that a well-designed insurance plan usually

FIGURE 3.1
The Flow of
Funds in
Healthcare
Markets

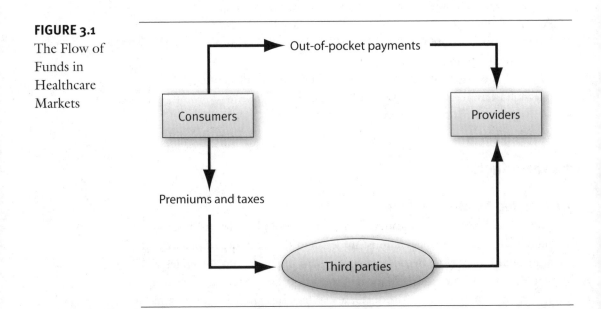

Sidebar 3.1 Boom and Bust in Home Care

The history of home care in the 1990s should be a warning to any manager whose business model relies on a single payer. Medicare home-care spending grew rapidly between 1989 and 1997. Visits per user nearly doubled, and the number of users increased sharply (Spector, Cohen, and Pesis-Katz 2004). There were several reasons for this boom. The introduction of the prospective payment system encouraged hospitals to discharge patients quickly to other settings, such as home care. Legal action in 1989 resulted in more generous eligibility and coverage, and new technology increased the number of patients who could receive adequate care at home. Some of the increased spending was for services of questionable value, and some was for services that were never delivered.

In 1997, however, the home-care boom halted abruptly. Exploding spending and stories of fraud prodded the government to act. The Balanced Budget Act of 1997 reduced payments and eligibility for home care and reduced incentives for hospitals to discharge patients to home care. In addition, Medicare took a number of steps to reduce fraud and abuse. The number of Medicare beneficiaries using home care fell by 20 percent, and visits per beneficiary fell by 40 percent. Home care spending fell sharply, and more than 10 percent of home care agencies went out of business. The boom was too good to be true, and a prudent manager would have anticipated a response by Medicare.

---

incorporates some cost sharing. We will explore this concept in detail in our discussion of demand in Chapter 6.

The extent of indirect payment in the healthcare market distinguishes it from most other markets. Indirect payment has three important functions:

1. It protects consumers against unexpectedly high healthcare expenses (one intention of third-party payers).
2. It encourages consumers to use additional healthcare services.
3. It limits the autonomy of consumers in healthcare decision making (not an intension of most third-party payers).

The advantages of indirect payment continue to exceed its disadvantages. As Chapter 2 showed, both the government and private insurance share of healthcare payments have increased substantially during the past 50 years.

3.1.3 The Uninsured

Most observers regard the rising number of uninsured as a problem. The percentage of the population without medical insurance rose from 12.9 percent in 1987 to 17.8 percent in 2006, even as out-of-pocket spending continued to fall as a share of total spending.

Uninsured consumers enter healthcare markets with two significant disadvantages. First, they must finance their needs from their own resources or the resources of family, friends, and well-wishers. If these funds are not adequate, they must do without care or rely on charity care. The uninsured do not have access to the vast resources of modern insurance companies when large healthcare bills arrive. Second, unlike most insured customers, uninsured customers may be expected to pay list prices for services. The majority of insured customers are covered by plans that have secured discounts from providers. For example, none of the major government insurance plans and few private insurance plans pay list prices for care. Although, in principle, uninsured patients could negotiate discounts on cash payments, this practice is not routine.

The uninsured tend to have low incomes. In 2007, 45 million Americans lacked health insurance. Sixty-five percent of them had family incomes below 200 percent of the federal poverty level (Holahan, Cook, and Dubay 2007). For many with low incomes, rising healthcare costs have made insurance unaffordable.

The combination of low income and no insurance often creates access problems. For example, in 2006, 25 percent of uninsured adults reported going without care due to cost, compared to 3 percent of privately insured adults. Likewise, 23 percent of uninsured adults reported not filling a prescription, compared to 4 percent of privately insured adults (Hoffman and Schwartz 2008). Delaying or forgoing care can lead to worse health outcomes.

Despite the continuing increase in the number of uninsured consumers, indirect payments continue to be the largest source of revenue for most healthcare providers. In 2006, they represented 97 percent of payments to hospitals, 89 percent of payments to physicians, and 74 percent of payments to nursing homes (Centers for Medicare & Medicaid Services 2008, Table 4). Because indirect payments are a factor in most healthcare purchases, their structure has a profound influence on the healthcare system and healthcare organizations.

3.2 What Is Insurance, and Why Is It So Prevalent?

3.2.1 What Insurance Does

Insurance pools the risks of healthcare costs, which have a skewed distribution. Most consumers have modest healthcare costs, but a few incur crushing sums. Insurance addresses this problem. Suppose that one person in a hundred will have the misfortune to run up $20,000 in healthcare bills. For simplicity, let's say no one else will have any healthcare bills. We can't predict who that unlucky person will be (or whether there will be an unlucky person at all), so consumers buy insurance so they have it in case they turn out to be that unlucky person. Let's say a private firm offers insurance for an annual premium of $240. Many consumers would be more than happy to pay $240 to eliminate a 1 percent chance of a $20,000 bill. (The extra $4,000 per 100 people the insurance firm earns would cover its selling costs, claims processing costs, and profits.)

3.2.2 Adverse Selection and Moral Hazard

Alas, the world is more complex than the preceding scenario, and such a simple plan probably would not work. To begin with, insurance tends to change the purchasing decisions of consumers. Insured consumers are more likely to use services, and providers no longer feel compelled to limit their diagnosis and treatment recommendations to amounts that individual consumers can afford. The increase in spending that occurs as a result of insurance coverage is known as *moral hazard.* Moral hazard can be substantially reduced if consumers face cost-sharing requirements, and most contemporary plans have this provision.

Another, less tractable problem remains. Some consumers, notably older people with chronic illnesses, are much more likely than average to face large bills. Such consumers would be especially eager to buy insurance. On the other hand, some consumers, notably younger people with healthy ancestors and no chronic illnesses, are much less likely than average to face large bills. Such consumers would not be especially eager to buy insurance. This situation illustrates *adverse selection*: people with high risk are eager to buy insurance, but people with low risk are not. At a minimum, the insurance firm would need to carefully assess the risks that individual consumers pose and base their premiums on those risks, a process known as *underwriting.* This process would drive up costs. In the worst case, no private firm would be willing to offer insurance to the general public.

In the United States, three mechanisms reduce the effects of adverse selection: employment-sponsored medical insurance, government-sponsored medical insurance, and medical insurance subsidies. In 2007, 85 percent of the population had medical insurance (DeNavas-Walt, Proctor, and Smith 2008). About 28 percent had government-sponsored medical insurance, and 57 percent had private medical insurance. (These figures count those with both government-sponsored and private insurance [as is the case with many Medicare beneficiaries] as having government-sponsored insurance.)

Virtually all Americans over age 65 have health insurance coverage through Medicare, a government insurance program. About 83 percent of those under age 65 have coverage, and most of them have private coverage (DeNavas-Walt, Proctor, and Smith 2008). Nine out of ten consumers with private insurance obtained it through their own or their spouse's employer.

Why is the link between employment and medical insurance so strong? To begin with, insurers are able to offer lower prices on employment-based insurance because they have cut their sales costs and their adverse selection risks by selling to groups. Selling a policy to a group of 1,000 people costs only a little more than selling a policy to an individual, thus the sales cost is much lower. And since few people take jobs or stay in them just because of the medical insurance benefits, adverse selection rarely occurs (i.e., all of the employees get the insurance, whether or not they think they'll need it soon). Medical insurance can also benefit employers. If coverage improves the health of employees or their dependents, workers will be more productive, thereby improving profits for the company. Companies also benefit because workers with employment-based medical insurance are less likely to quit. The costs of hiring and training employees are high, so firms do not want to lose employees unnecessarily.

The most salient factor in the link between employment and medical insurance is the substantial tax savings that employment-based medical insurance provides. Medical insurance provided as a benefit is excluded from Social Security taxes, Medicare taxes, federal income taxes, and most state and local income taxes. Earning $4,000 in cash instead of a $4,000 medical insurance benefit could easily increase an employee's tax bill by $2,000.

This system is clearly advantageous from the perspective of insurers, employers, and employees. From the perspective of society as a whole, however, its desirability is less clear. The subsidies built into the tax code tend to force tax rates higher, may encourage insurance for "uninsurable" costs like eyeglasses and routine dental checkups, and give employees an unrealistic sense of how much insurance costs.

Another disadvantage is found in the way most employers frame health insurance benefits. In 2007, less than 15 percent of private employers allowed employees to choose between plans (Kaiser Family Foundation 2007a). Larger employers were more likely to offer a choice of plans. In addition, most employers pay more when an employee selects a more expensive plan, which gives them little incentive to offer one. Few employers share information about the quality of care offered through different plans or other aspects of plan performance. Without this information, employees are unlikely to be able to identify plans with better provider networks or better customer service.

3.2.3 Medicare as an Example of Complexity

The health insurance system in the United States is so complex that only a few specialists understand it. Figure 3.2 illustrates the complexity of healthcare financing, even in simple cases. To demonstrate this complexity,

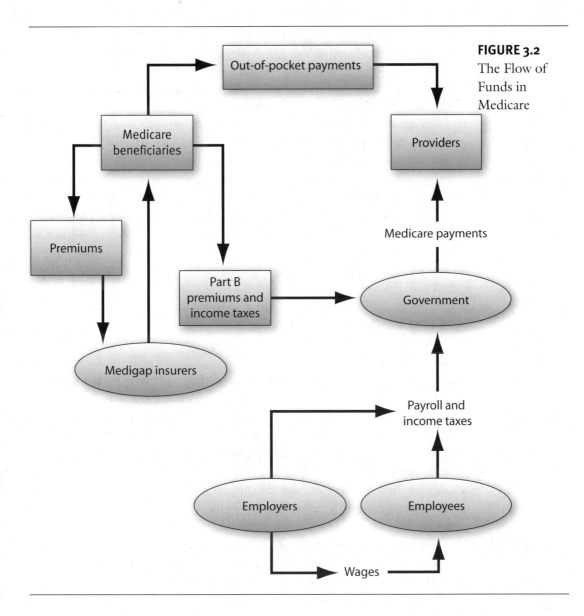

FIGURE 3.2
The Flow of Funds in Medicare

we will examine the flow of funds in Medicare, starting with Medicare beneficiaries. Many pay premiums for Medigap policies that cover deductibles, coinsurance, and other expenses that Medicare does not cover. Like many insurers, Medicare requires a deductible. In 2007, the Part A deductible was $992 per year and the Part B deductible was $131. The most common coinsurance payments spring from the 20 percent of allowed fees Medicare beneficiaries must pay for most Part B services. To keep Figure 3.2 simple, we have focused on Medigap policies that reimburse beneficiaries rather than pay providers directly. Beneficiaries with these sorts of policies (and many without Medigap coverage) must make required out-of-pocket payments directly to providers. Beneficiaries must also pay the Part B premiums that fund 25 percent of this Medicare component. Like other taxpayers, beneficiaries must also pay income taxes that cover the other 75 percent of Part B costs.

Employers and employees also pay taxes to fund the Medicare system. The most visible of these taxes is the Medicare payroll tax, which is levied on wages to fund Part A (which covers hospital, home health, skilled nursing, and hospice services). In addition, corporation and individual income taxes help fund the 75 percent of Part B costs that premiums do not cover. The Centers for Medicare & Medicaid Services, the federal agency that operates Medicare, combines these tax and premium funds to pay providers. Not surprisingly, few taxpayers, beneficiaries, and public officials understand how Medicare is financed.

3.3 The Rise of Managed Care

Traditional open-ended fee-for-service plans (of which pre-1984 Medicare was a classic example) have three basic problems. First, they encourage providers and consumers to use covered services as long as the direct cost to consumers is less than the direct benefit. Because the actual total cost of care is much greater than consumers pay, some may use services that are not worth as much as they actually cost. In addition, open-ended fee-for-service plans discourage consumers from using services that are not covered, even highly effective ones. Finally, much of the system is unplanned, in that the prices paid by consumers and the prices received by providers do not reflect actual provider costs or consumer valuations.

Given the origins of traditional medical insurance, this inattention to efficiency makes sense. Medical insurance was started by providers, largely in response to consumers' inability to afford expensive services and the unwillingness of some consumers to pay their bills once services had been rendered. The goal was to cover the costs of services, not to provide care in the most efficient manner possible and not to improve the health of the covered population.

Managed care is a collection of insurance plans with only one common denominator: a perception that traditional, open-ended, fee-for-service (FFS) insurance plans are no longer tenable. A traditional open-ended plan covered all services if they were covered by the contract and if a provider, typically a physician, was willing to certify that they were medically necessary. Payment to the provider was based on submitted charges, so hospital care was "free" from the perspective of physicians. In many cases, hospital care did not cost patients very much either. Generous coverage of hospital ser-

Case 3.1

Should the Federal Employees Health Benefits Program Be a Model?

Many Americans have little choice about health insurance. For the majority, the choices are to accept the plan offered by their employer, by their state Medicaid agency, or by Medicare, or to do without. Even Americans who have a choice lack the information needed to choose wisely. In many respects, the Federal Employees Health Benefits Program is superior. Its structure reflects the concept of managed competition first advocated by Stanford University economist Alain Enthoven (1984):

- Each year employees choose one of several private insurance plans.
- The government pays the same amount regardless of the employee's choice. If the government pays $3,000 per year, the employee pays $1,000 if she chooses a plan costing $4,000, and pays $2,000 if she chooses a plan costing $5,000.
- Insurance providers must accept everyone and must charge everyone the same premium.

This structure would inject choice, competition, and cost consciousness into insurance choices.

How has it worked? Compared to private employer plan premiums, federal plan premiums have risen more slowly in some years and have risen more rapidly in others (U.S. Government Accountability Office 2006). The overall pattern, however, is similar to the patterns of other private insurer plan premiums.

One difficulty is that competition is largely for good risks. High-cost plans tend to serve populations that are likely to spend a lot on medical care, and low-cost plans tend to serve populations that are likely to spend little. The simplest, fastest way for an insurer to increase profits and market share is to discourage a few customers who are likely to incur high costs and to recruit customers who are likely to incur low costs. Not surprisingly, insurance plans tend to emphasize good access to primary care services, not good access to cancer or cardiac specialists (who will be used by patients who spend a lot). Healthcare spending is highly skewed, so 20 percent of the population accounts for 80 percent of spending (Kaiser Family Foundation 2007b). Avoiding even a few high-cost patients can dramatically improve an insurer's profitability. Furthermore, many consumers change plans every few years, so investing in preventive services may not make sense for insurers. The federal plan should make employees focus on differences in insurance costs, but the insurers serving this population have not been unusually innovative in finding new ways to bring down costs.

(continued)

vices and limited coverage of some outpatient services meant that extensive use of costly hospital services served the needs of patients and physicians well but drove healthcare costs higher and higher.

At present, managed care takes four basic forms: preferred provider organizations (PPOs), staff and group model health maintenance organizations (HMOs), independent-practice association (IPA) HMOs, and point-of-service HMOs. We will briefly describe each of these forms of managed care organizations.

PPOs are the most common form of managed care organization. All PPOs negotiate discounts with a panel of hospitals, physicians, and other providers, but their similarities end there. Some PPOs have small panels; others have large panels. Some PPOs require that care be approved by a primary care physician; some do not.

PPOs are far less diverse than HMOs, however. Traditional HMOs are structured around large group practices. Group model HMOs contract with a small number of groups; staff model HMOs employ physicians directly. Group model HMOs usually capitate payment to physician groups (i.e., they pay physicians per consumer enrolled with them). Staff model HMOs usually pay salaries. These HMOs still exist, but they are expensive to set up and make sense only for large numbers of enrollees. HMO expansion largely has been fueled by the growth of IPA HMOs. These plans contract with large groups of physicians, small groups of physicians, and solo practice physicians. These contracts assume many forms. Physicians can be paid per service (as PPOs usually operate) or per enrollee (as group model HMOs usually operate). IPAs also pay hospitals and other providers in different ways.

The point-of-service (POS) plan is another form of HMO. These plans are a combination of PPO and IPA. Unlike an IPA, they cover nonemergency services provided by nonnetwork providers, but copayments are higher. Unlike a PPO, they pay some providers using methods other than discounted fee-for-service.

Managed care continues to evolve in a disorderly fashion. Where this development will lead is not clear. There is widespread belief that managed care is in retreat, but Figure 3.3 indicates otherwise. The market share of fee-for-service plans has continued to fall, and the market share of PPO plans has continued to rise. HMO plans have lost market share, likely attributable to the fact that PPO plans do not cost much more, are easier to operate, and are better accepted by consumers.

Managed care plans seek to change the incentives open-ended fee-for-service plans create. Some managed care plans seek to change financial incentives for providers. Medicare's diagnosis-related group (DRG) system and the global payment systems of some HMOs are examples of this shift. Other managed care plans seek to change financial incentives for consumers. Lower copayments for preventive services and higher copayments for branded pharmaceuticals are examples of this shift toward consumer incentive.

Some managed care plans seek to use their market power to secure advantageous contracts. Most plans negotiate provider discounts. Other managed care plans seek to create bureaucratic structures, commonly called *utilization review plans*, that reduce the use of low-value care and increase the use of high-value care.

Still other managed care plans seek to select providers with below-average costs and above-average outcomes. All of these sorts of arrangements are most common in tightly integrated plans, which contract with a limited number of hospitals and physician groups. In turn, the physician groups deal with a limited number of insurance plans. In the most tightly integrated plans, physicians treat only patients covered by one plan. Typically, physicians treat patients insured by hundreds of plans.

3.3.1 How Do Insurance Plans Manage Care?

What did managed care plans do to alter patterns of care that traditional insurance plans did not? Less than you might imagine, according to several studies (Remler et al. 1997; Kapur, Gresenz, and Studdert 2003). In the

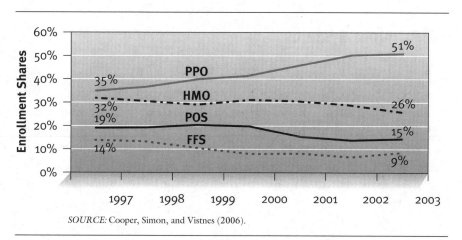

FIGURE 3.3
Insurance Enrollment Patterns

SOURCE: Cooper, Simon, and Vistnes (2006).

1990s, managed care plans often required prior authorization of some types of care and denied coverage for unauthorized services that were not deemed emergency care. Managed care plans also denied coverage for services not in their networks of hospitals and physicians. There is no evidence that denials of coverage exceeded 10 percent, and as many as three-fourths of initial denials were overturned if beneficiaries appealed (Kapur, Gresenz, and Studdert 2003). The net effect, therefore, was to increase the administrative burdens on providers and patients, which created a significant backlash, without significantly reducing costs.

Not surprisingly, therefore, insurers have moved away from models of the 1990s in many areas. Networks tend to be larger, and use of non-network providers simply costs patients a bit more. Indeed, many of the new tools involve fairly simple financial incentives. These include lower patient costs for highly effective interventions (such as proven medications for patients with chronic conditions), higher patient costs for interventions that do not appear to be cost effective (such as expensive branded drugs with inexpensive generic alternatives), and bonuses for physicians who meet standards of care (Chernew, Rosen, and Fendrick 2007). Such an approach encourages, but does not require, physicians and patients to do what the insurer thinks is appropriate. The hope is that this will reduce costs and improve quality without inciting a backlash.

Yet some older models of managed care continue to flourish. The number of radiology benefits managers, most of whom manage prior approvals of imaging services, has grown rapidly in recent years. In fact, a recent report suggested that Medicare consider emulating this system of prior approvals for imaging services (U.S. Government Accountability Office 2008). Medicare spending for imaging more than doubled between 2000 to 2006, and in 2008 Congress mandated a test of prior approvals for Medicare imaging. The search for new ways to manage care continues.

3.4 Payment Systems

In the past, most healthcare providers were paid on a simple fee-for-service basis. Today, managed care plans have begun to experiment with alternative payment arrangements. Different payment systems are important because they create different incentive systems for providers. Differences in financial incentives lead to different patterns of care, so the power of changing incentives should not be underestimated. In contracting with insurers or providers, managers need to recognize the strengths and weaknesses of different systems.

Case 3.2 The Fourth Tier in Pharmaceutical Coverage

Most insurers have adopted tiered formularies that cover most drugs approved by the Food and Drug Administration. Tier 1 charges the lowest copayments or coinsurance and includes most generic drugs. (Generic drugs are developed when brand-name drugs' patents expire. They contain the same active ingredients as their corresponding brand-name drugs. For example, Sulfasalazine is the generic version of Azulfidine, a medication for patients with ulcerative colitis. The list price of Sulfasalazine is about 25 percent the price of Azulfidine.) Tier 2 drugs are more expensive than tier 1 drugs. Most are brand-name products with branded or generic alternatives. Tier 3 drugs cost more than tier 2 drugs and include branded drugs the insurer has not included in tier 2.

This approach has several advantages. First, it gives patients an incentive to use generic or inexpensive brand-name medications. Second, it lets physicians and patients choose any drug the patient is willing to pay for. Third, it gives insurers leverage in negotiating discounts in exchange for including a branded product in tier 2 (in which its sales will be much higher than if it were limited to tier 3).

Recently a new tier has been added to some plans. Tier 4 drugs are more expensive than the drugs in tiers 1–3, and many do not have branded or generic alternatives. Medicare drug plans introduced this tier, and other plans are beginning to include it. Patients are often expected to pay 20–35 percent of the cost of tier 4 drugs. For example, a patient with hepatitis C would be expected to pay between $150 and $210 per dose of Intron A. Patients who have been prescribed a tier 4 drug have four options: absorb the cost, switch to another medication, disregard the prescription, or switch to another insurance plan. Any of these options would reduce the insurer's costs, often substantially, and allow the insurer to keep premiums low.

Some observers strongly object to plans with four tiers. For example, James Robinson, a health economist at the University of California, noted that a tier 4 plan could stick seriously ill people with huge bills (Kolata 2008). Others have objected that plans with four tiers undermine the fundamental principles of insurance. Yet, at a time when some drug therapies can cost $100,000 per year for modest health benefits, plans with four tiers remain an option for keeping costs down.

Discussion questions:
- How would the options open to patients who have been prescribed a tier 4 drug affect their insurers' costs? The patients' costs?
- Suppose you are an insurer and a competing insurer implemented a fourth tier and you did not. What would happen to their costs and yours? How would you respond? What does this scenario tell you about competition between insurers?
- Do you think plans with four tiers should be permitted? Explain your answer.

The four basic payment methods—salary, fee-for-service, case-based, and capitation—can be modified by the addition of incentive payments, increasing the number of possible payment methods.

A *salary* is fixed compensation paid per defined period. As such, it is not directly linked to output. Typically, physicians are paid a salary when their productivity is difficult to measure (e.g., in the case of academic physicians) or when the incentives created by fee-for-service payments are seen as undesirable (e.g., an incentive to overtreat increases costs). As stated earlier, most physicians in the United States have traditionally been paid on a *fee-for-service* basis, meaning each physician has a schedule of fees and expects to be paid that amount for each unit of service provided.

Case-based payments make single payments for all covered services associated with an episode of care. Medicare's DRG system is a case-based system for hospital care, although it does not include physicians' services or post-hospital care. In essence, case-based payments are fee-for-service payments for a wider range of services. *Capitation* is compensation paid per beneficiary enrolled with a physician or an organization. Capitation is similar to a salary but varies according to the number of customers.

Each of the four basic payment methods has advantages and disadvantages. Salaries are straightforward and incorporate no incentives to provide more care than necessary, but they do not encourage outstanding effort or exemplary service. In addition, salaries give providers incentives to use resources other than their time and effort to meet their customers' needs. In the absence of incentives not to, salaried providers may well seek to refer substantial numbers of patients to specialists, urgent care clinics, or other sources of care.

Capitation incorporates many of the same incentives as a salary, except there are two important differences. One is that capitation payments drop if customers defect, so physicians have more incentive to serve patients well. The other is that capitation arrangements often generate extra costs. Profits rise if these extra costs fall, so capitation encourages greater efficiency, referral to other providers, or insufficient treatment.

In contrast, fee-for-service payments create powerful incentives to provide superior service, so much that overtreatment of insured consumers often results. Services that are more costly than beneficial can be profitable in this system, as long as the benefits exceed the consumer's out-of-pocket cost. These incentives can complicate efforts to control costs. For example, attempts to impose or negotiate lower rates are likely to provoke providers to "unbundle" care by billing separately for procedures or tests that had been combined as one service.

The case-based method combines features of the fee-for-service and capitation methods. Like fee-for-service, it creates strong incentives to provide exceptional service, as well as an additional incentive to increase profits

Case 3.3   Aetna's Retreat from Managed Care

The managed care era assumed that high healthcare costs resulted from unnecessary use of services, high prices for services, and high administrative costs. The growing evidence of variability in prices and utilization (and insufficient evidence that high prices or high levels of service produce better patient outcomes) is consistent with this view (Wennberg 2004). Furthermore, there is considerable evidence that administrative costs (which contribute little to patient outcomes) are high in the current system (Woolhandler, Campbell, and Himmelstein 2003). These assumptions appear to have been correct, yet something of a retreat from managed care seems to be under way.

The history of Aetna illustrates this retreat (Robinson 2004). Circa 1990 Aetna was a conservative, profitable commercial carrier focused on fee-for-service coverage of employees and retirees of large, self-insured corporations. Aetna steered clear of the individual insurance market and most forms of managed care. Yet Aetna moved aggressively into managed care, paying a hefty price to merge with U. S. Healthcare (a major HMO insurer) in 1996, acquiring Prudential Healthcare in 1998, and acquiring NYL Healthcare in 1999.

By 2000, however, investors forced the resignation of Richard L. Huber, the CEO who orchestrated this transformation. In short order, Aetna deemphasized the HMO contracts its new acquisitions had emphasized and focused on other products. Although Aetna continued to negotiate discounts, the company had largely reverted to its earlier, minimally intrusive approach. Aetna's retreat from aggressive managed care and renewed focus on profitability led to a rapid improvement in earnings. Its days as an HMO were over. Although Aetna still offers what it calls "network-only" plans, the company focuses on flexible plans that are easy to use and have features customers want (Thomson Business Intelligence Service 2006). It even offers old-fashioned indemnity plans that allow customers to see any licensed provider.

The company is currently pushing to improve the quality of care for customers with multiple chronic conditions because, as Troyen Brennan, Aetna's chief medical officer noted, "that's where the money is and that's where the bad healthcare is" (Thomson Business Intelligence Service 2006). Modest improvements in the care of seriously ill patients, who account for at least 80 percent of medical costs, can significantly reduce costs. For example, using its data, Aetna can identify customers who have had a heart attack and the medications they take. If those medications stray from the regimen suggested by the best available clinical evidence, Aetna contacts the customer and his or her physician. Alerting the beneficiary and physician to potential problems has reduced hospitalizations by over 8 percent, a significant savings (Thomson Business Intelligence Service 2006).

(continued)

by reducing costs included in the case rate. Costs can be reduced by
improving efficiency, shifting responsibility for therapy to "free" sources
(such as the heath department), and narrowing the definition of a case. The
challenge is to keep providers focused on improving efficiency, not on dup-
ing the system.

Any of these four basic methods can be modified by including
bonuses and penalties. A base salary plus a bonus for reducing inpatient
days in selected cases is not a straight salary contract. Similarly, a capitation
plan with bonuses or penalties for exceeding or not meeting customer service standards (e.g., a bonus for returning more than 75 percent of after-
hours calls within 15 minutes) would not generate the same incentives a
plain capitation plan would.

Capitation had been expected to become the dominant method of
payment. Experience with capitation suggests, however, that few providers
(or insurers, for that matter) have the administrative skills or data that capitation demands. In addition, the financial risks of capitation can be substantial. Few providers have enough capitated patients for variations in average
costs to cease being worrisome, and capitation payments are seldom risk
adjusted (i.e., increased when spending can be expected to be higher than

average). These considerations have dampened most providers' enthusiasm for capitation. Insurers also have realized that capitation is not a panacea, recognizing that providers have ways other than becoming more efficient to reduce their costs. At present, fee-for-service payments to providers remain the norm, even in most HMOs. What compensation arrangements will look like in ten years remains to be seen.

3.5 Conclusion

The days of traditional, open-ended insurance plans are over. Even plans that are not called managed care plans usually have incorporated some managed care components to keep premiums down. Despite managed care plans' market takeover, however, most consumers are enrolled in plans that are minimally managed, such as PPO or POS plans that pay providers in familiar ways, and most providers are not part of an organized delivery system.

Dramatic changes in spending are also evident. Consumers' direct spending continues to drop, even as the proportion of consumers without health insurance continues to rise. Coverage of those with insurance has become more comprehensive, and tax-financed spending has continued to rise. Cost sharing by patients has become a routine part of health insurance plans while use of other forms of direct spending has declined.

The process of change substantially increases the risks healthcare managers must face. The next chapter will introduce the basics of how to manage these risks.

Homework

3.1   Why is health insurance necessary?

3.2   Explain how adverse selection and moral hazard are different, and give an example of each.

3.3   "The United States is the land of the overinsured, the underinsured, and the uninsured." What do you think these concepts mean? Why might this comment be true?

3.4   Private health insurers have been slow to develop and adopt proven cost containment innovations (e.g., case rates or disease management programs). Why do you think this is the case?

3.5   A radiology firm charges $2,000 per exam. Uninsured patients are expected to pay list price. How much do they pay?

3.6   A radiology firm charges $2,000 per exam. An insurer's allowed fee is 80 percent of charges. Its beneficiaries pay 25 percent of the allowed fee. How much does the insurer pay? How much does the beneficiary pay?

3.7   If the radiology firm raised its charge to $3,000, how much would the insurer pay? How much would the beneficiary pay?

3.8   A surgeon charges $2,400 for hernia surgery. He contracts with an insurer that allows a fee of $800. Patients pay 20 percent of the allowed fee. How much does the insurer pay? How much does the patient pay?

3.9   You have incurred a medical bill of $10,000. Your plan has a deductible of $1,000 and coinsurance of 20 percent. How much of this bill will you have to pay directly?

3.10   Why do employers provide health insurance coverage to their employees?

3.11   Your practice offers only a PPO with a large deductible, high coinsurance, and a limited network. You pay $400 per month for single coverage. Some of your employees have been urging you to offer a more generous plan. Who would you expect to choose the more generous plan and pay any extra premium?

3.12   What are the fundamental differences between HMO and PPO plans?

3.13   Suppose that your employer offered you $4,000 in cash instead of health insurance coverage. Health insurance is excluded from state income taxes and federal income taxes. (To keep the problem simple, we will ignore Social Security and Medicare taxes.) The cash would be subject to state income taxes (8%), and federal income taxes (28%). How much would your after-tax income go up if you took the cash rather than insurance?

3.14   How different would this calculation look for a worker who earned $500,000 and lived in Vermont? This worker would face a federal income tax rate of 35 percent and a state income tax rate of 9.5 percent.

Chapter Glossary

Adverse selection. High-risk consumers' willingness to pay more for insurance than low-risk consumers (Organizations that have difficulty distinguishing high-risk from low-risk consumers are unlikely to be profitable.)

Capitation. Payment per person (The payment does not depend on the services provided.)

Case-based payment. A single payment for an episode of care (The payment does not change if fewer services or more services are provided.)

Coinsurance. A form of cost sharing in which a patient pays a share of the bill rather than a set fee

Copayment. A fee the patient must pay in addition to the amount paid by insurance

Cost sharing. The general term for direct payments to providers by insurance beneficiaries (Deductibles, copayments, and coinsurance are forms of cost sharing.)

Diagnosis-related groups (DRGs). Case groups that underlie Medicare's case-based payment system for hospitals

Fee-for-service. An insurance plan that pays providers on the basis of their charges for services

Formulary. A formulary can be a list of drugs routinely used by a healthcare provider, or it can be a list of prescription drugs covered by insurance.

Group model HMO. HMO that contracts with a physician group to provide services

Health maintenance organization (HMO). A firm that provides comprehensive healthcare benefits to enrollees in exchange for a premium (Originally, HMOs were distinct from other insurance firms because providers were not paid on a fee-for-service basis and because enrollees faced no cost-sharing requirements.)

Managed care. A loosely defined term that includes PPO and HMO plans, sometimes used to describe the techniques insurance companies use

Medicaid. The name given to a collection of state programs that meet standards set by the Centers for Medicare & Medicaid Services but run by state agencies (Medicaid serves those with incomes low enough to qualify for their state's program.)

Medicare. An insurance program for the elderly and disabled that is run by the Centers for Medicare & Medicaid Services

Medicare Part A. Coverage for inpatient hospital, skilled nursing, hospice, and home healthcare services

Medicare Part B. Coverage for outpatient services and medical equipment

Moral hazard. The incentive to use additional care that having insurance creates

Point-of-service (POS) plan. Plan that allows members to see any physician but increases cost sharing for physicians outside the plan's network (This arrangement has become so common that POS plans may not be labeled as such.)

Preferred provider organization (PPO). An insurance plan that contracts with a network of providers (Network providers may be chosen for a

variety of reasons, but a willingness to discount fees is usually
required.)

Staff model HMO. HMO that directly employs staff physicians to provide
services

Underwriting. The process of assessing the risks associated with an
insurance policy and setting the premium accordingly

Utilization review. Analysis of patterns of resource use

References

Centers for Medicare & Medicaid Services. 2008. "National Health Expenditures, by
Source of Funds and Type of Expenditure." [Online information; retrieved
3/13/08.] www.cms.hhs.gov/NationalHealthExpendData/downloads/
tables.pdf.

Chernew, M. E., A. B. Rosen, and A. M. Fendrick. 2007. "Value-Based Insurance
Design." *Health Affairs* 26 (2): w195–w203.

Cooper, P. F., K. I. Simon, and J. Vistnes. 2006. "A Closer Look at the Managed
Care Backlash." *Medical Care* 44 (5, Suppl.): I4–11.

DeNavas-Walt, C., B. D. Proctor, and J. C. Smith. 2008. "Current Population
Reports, P60–235, Income, Poverty, and Health Insurance Coverage in
the United States: 2007." U.S. Census Bureau. [Online information;
retrieved 11/19/08.] www.census.gov/prod/2008pubs/p60–235.pdf.

Enthoven, A. 1984. "A New Proposal to Reform the Tax Treatment of Health
Insurance." *Health Affairs* 3 (1): 21–39.

Gruber, J. 2006. "The Role of Consumer Copayments for Health Care: Lessons
from the RAND Health Insurance Experiment and Beyond." [Online
information; retrieved 3/21/08.] www.kff.org/insurance/upload/
7566.pdf.

Hoffman, C., and K. Schwartz. 2008. "Trends in Access to Care Among Working-
Age Adults." [Online information; retrieved 11/19/08.] www.kff.org.

Holahan, J., A. Cook, and L. Dubay. 2007. *Characteristics of the Uninsured: Who Is
Eligible for Public Coverage and Who Needs Help Affording Coverage?*
[Online information; retrieved 11/19/08.] www.kff.org/uninsured/
upload/7613.pdf.

Kaiser Family Foundation. 2007a. *Employer Health Benefits 2007.* [Online
information; retrieved 3/23/08.] www.kff.org/insurance.

Kaiser Family Foundation. 2007b. "Trends in Health Care Costs and Spending."
    [Online information; retrieved 3/14/08. www.kff.org/insurance/upload/
    7692.pdf.

Kapur, K., C. R. Gresenz, and D. M. Studdert. 2003. "Managing Care: Utilization
    Review in Action at Two Capitated Medical Groups." *Health Affairs Web
    Exclusive*: W3–275–282. [Online information; retrieved 11/22/08.]
    http://content.healthaffairs.org/cgi/content/full/hlthaff.w3.275v1/DC1.

Kolata, G. 2008. "Co-Payments Soar for Drugs with High Prices." [Online
    information; retrieved 4/16/08.] http://nytimes.com.

Remler, D. K., K. Donelan, R. J. Blendon, G. D. Lundberg, L. L. Leape, D. R.
    Calkins, K. Binns, and J. P. Newhouse. 1997. "What Do Managed Care
    Plans Do to Affect Care? Results from a Survey of Physicians." *Inquiry*
    34 (3): 196–204.

Robinson, J. C. 2004. "From Managed Care to Consumer Health Insurance: The
    Fall and Rise of Aetna." *Health Affairs* 23 (2): 43–55.

Robinson, J. C., and J. M. Yegian. 2004. "Medical Management After Managed
    Care." *Health Affairs Web Exclusive*. [Online information; retrieved
    11/25/08.] http://content.healthaffairs.org/cgi/content/full/
    hlthaff.w4.269v1/DC1.

Spector, W. D., J. W. Cohen, and I. Pesis-Katz. 2004. "Home Care Before and
    After the Balanced Budget Act of 1997: Shifts in Financing and Services."
    The Gerontologist 44 (1): 39–48.

Thomson Business Intelligence Service. 2006. "Aetna Inc. Analyst Meeting."
    [Online information; retrieved 3/23/08.] http://insurancenewsnet.com.

U.S. Government Accountability Office. 2006. "Federal Employees Health Benefits
    Program." [Online information; retrieved 3/14/08.] www.gao.gov/
    new.items/d07141.pdf.

———. 2008. "Medicare Part B Imaging Services." [Online information; retrieved
    11/25/08.] www.gao.gov/new.items/d08452.pdf.

Wennberg, J. E. 2004. "Perspective: Practice Variations and Health Care Reform:
    Connecting the Dots." [Online information; retrieved 3/21/08.]
    www.healthaffairs.org.

Woolhandler, S., T. Campbell, and D. U. Himmelstein. 2003. "Costs of Health
    Care Administration in the United States and Canada." *New England
    Journal of Medicine* 349 (8): 768–75.

DESCRIBING, EVALUATING, AND MANAGING RISK

Learning Objectives

After reading this chapter, students will be able to:

- **calculate** an expected value and standard deviation,
- **describe** the key features of a risky outcome,
- **construct and use** a decision tree to frame a choice, and
- **discuss** common approaches to managing risk.

Key Concepts

- Clinical and managerial decisions typically entail uncertainty about what will happen.
- Decision makers often have imprecise estimates of the probabilities of various outcomes.
- Decision making about risk involves describing, evaluating, and managing potential outcomes.
- Insurance and diversification are two ways to manage risk.

4.1 Introduction

Clinical and managerial decisions typically entail risk. Important information is often incomplete or missing when the time to make a decision arrives. At best, one is aware of potential outcomes and the probability of each outcome's occurrence. At worst, one has little to no information about outcomes and their probabilities. The challenge for managers is to identify risks that are worth analyzing, risks that are worth taking, and the best strategy for dealing with them.

When outcomes are uncertain, decision making has three components: describing, evaluating, and managing potential outcomes. Because uncertainty is central to many areas of healthcare, the same techniques (e.g., hedging bets and aggressive monitoring of uncertain situations) are recommended for describing and evaluating potential outcomes regarding real investments (e.g., buildings, equipment, and training), financial investments (e.g., stocks, bonds, and insurance), and clinical decisions (e.g., testing and therapy).

4.2 Describing Potential Outcomes

The first step in any decision is to describe what could happen, including the probabilities and value of possible outcomes, and to calculate descriptive statistics about them.

Description begins with an assessment of the probabilities of the possible outcomes. Ideally, these probabilities should be objective—based on evidence about the frequencies of different outcomes. For example, if 250 of 1,000 patients reported nausea after taking a medication, a good estimate of the probability of nausea would be 0.25 (250 divided by 1,000). More often though, description assesses subjective probabilities—the decision maker's perception of how likely an outcome will occur.

In some cases, decision makers have incomplete data. In other cases, the data do not fit. For example, if a careful study of a drug in a population of men over age 18 finds that the probability of nausea is 0.25, what value should we use for a sample of women over age 65? In still other cases, individuals may feel that population frequencies do not apply to them. Someone who claims to have a "cast-iron stomach" may believe that his probability of nausea is much less than 0.25. The decision maker with a "cast-iron stomach" may be correct in thinking that the population frequencies do not apply to him or he may just be overly optimistic.

In practice, decision makers predominantly use subjective probabilities. Unfortunately, these subjective probabilities are often inaccurate, even when made by highly trained clinicians or experienced managers. Studies have found that physicians overestimate the probability of skull fractures, cancer, pneumonia, and streptococcal infections, and managers are notorious for being overenthusiastic in their forecasts of how well new projects will be run and how well they will be received. For a variety of reasons, humans generally are poor probability calculators. Examining data about population frequencies can significantly improve decision makers' choices. For example, even if you believe that your hospital is less likely than average to lose money on the primary care practices it has just purchased, knowing that the majority of hospitals have lost money tells you that you are still prone to loss. Moreover, in many cases, an honest assessment of the probabilities results in broad generalizations, not a point estimate of probabilities. A manager may be able to say only that he or she thinks one scenario is more likely than another. This information is still useful; general impressions can often clarify the situation and help managers make the best decision.

Case 4.1   Betting on Medicare Advantage

Risk is intrinsic to the health insurance business. Insurers take on risk by selling coverage for consumers' variable medical expenditures. When you average risk over the spending patterns of tens of thousands of consumers, however, it becomes less uncertain—in most cases. In 2008, Humana nearly halved its profit forecast because claims for its Medicare prescription drug plan ran much higher than anticipated. Apparently, its emphasis on covering well-known, branded pharmaceuticals attracted a large number of customers with above-average utilization patterns. (This situation is an example of adverse selection.)

But the real risks do not come from operations issues such as those mentioned above. The real risks spring from strategic decisions that could result in great loss or problems if an insurer misjudges the market or if the market takes a sudden turn. For example, Humana's decision to serve Medicare Advantage customers in 2007 was a major gamble. From one perspective, it looks like a safe bet. The number of potential customers will continue to increase steadily for years to come, and Medicare Advantage rates are high enough to make them profitable customers.

The problem is that these high rates make Medicare Advantage an obvious political target. Estimates are that Medicare Advantage plans cost taxpayers 12 percent more than traditional Medicare (Congressional Budget Office 2007). The initial gamble is that the 110th Congress will do nothing to reduce rates, even though a number of bills to cut rates were filed in 2007. The next gamble is that the new president and new Congress in 2009 will not take steps to make Medicare Advantage an unattractive business. Other insurers perceive the risk in serving Medicare Advantage customers as too high. For example, WellPoint, Aetna, and CIGNA have been reluctant to invest in this market, wary of potential changes in federal rules or payments. And all of these companies are facing the slowdown of the private health insurance market.

Discussion questions:

- What has happened to Medicare Advantage since the spring of 2008?
- Was Humana's bet a good one, or was the caution of CIGNA the better call?
- Medicare Advantage contracts last a year. What is Humana risking by betting that Medicare Advantage will be an attractive opportunity?
- What else could Humana have done to manage the risks associated with Medicare Advantage?
- Is Medicare Advantage riskier than other parts of private health insurance? Explain your answer.
- Are other healthcare firms also subject to risks associated with changes in government policy? Can you offer examples of firms that are or are not at risk?

4.3 Evaluating Outcomes

The next step is to evaluate possible outcomes. This chapter focuses on financial outcomes, typically profits. Financial outcomes are usually difficult to project. Skilled analysts commonly arrive at different answers when asked to calculate how much a therapy will cost under well-defined circumstances. Attempts at forecasting costs and revenues for a new project result in an even greater range of plausible outcomes because of all the attendant uncertainties inherent in such an undertaking. Analysts may have ways of improving their forecasts, but in general, forecasts will never be more than educated guesses.

As you can imagine, the problems mount when no simple measurement system, like profits, exists. How valuable is a new surgical procedure that reduces the chance of abdominal scarring from 0.12 to 0.08 but reduces the chance that the operation will succeed from 0.68 to 0.66? Any time a scenario involves opposing probabilities, evaluation becomes a challenge. Even though scholars have made progress in evaluating complex outcomes, considerable uncertainty remains. Chapter 13 will tackle this problem in more detail.

Calculating descriptive statistics is the final step in the process of evaluating outcomes. The most common statistic is the expected value. To calculate an expected value, multiply the value of each outcome by its probability of occurrence and then add the resulting products. For example, suppose your organization is contemplating buying a skilled nursing facility that currently has profits of $20,000. The price of the nursing home is $1 million, meaning that the return on investment would be only 2 percent, which is too low from your organization's point of view. (Return on investment equals annual profit divided by your investment.) One of your managers, however, has identified a number of operational improvements that she forecasts will boost profits to $120,000. Although this manager's improvements are reasonable, a consultant points out that, in his experience, ambitious proposals to increase profits fail about 40 percent of the time. So, the consultant estimates that the expected profit is $80,000 = (0.6 × $120,000) + (0.4 × $20,000).

This level of precision (e.g., "about 40 percent of the time") is representative of the reliability of managerial forecasts—they are inexact at best. Despite imprecise forecasts, managers must make a choice. In many cases, calculating the expected profit and then conducting a sensitivity analysis will help managers avoid bad decisions.

Formally, an expected value equals $P_1X_1 + P_2X_2 + \ldots + P_nX_n$, where P_i represents the probability that an outcome will occur and X_i represents the value of that outcome. An expected value differs from an average because the probabilities of some outcomes will be higher than the probabilities of others, so they get more weight. For example, the average of

$120,000 and $20,000—the two estimates from our example above—is $70,000. But the expected value is $80,000 because the probability of earning $120,000 is larger than the probability of earning $20,000.

Does buying the skilled nursing home make sense? It might. Expected return on investment is 8 percent. Given that the worst-case scenario is a 2 percent return on investment, this gamble will seem reasonable to many firms, depending on the alternative investments the firm is considering.

Good decisions usually require more information than just an expected value because typically the expected value is not the outcome that occurs. Most decision makers find that a list of the best and worst outcomes is valuable. A list of the most likely outcomes can also be useful. Graphs, too, can help decision makers understand their choices. Many people find a well-designed graph more valuable than a calculation. Finally, remember that estimates are estimates; writing them down does not make them more reliable. The less mathematically sophisticated your target audience is, the more you need to emphasize that forecasts are imprecise.

This simple example can be illustrated with a *decision tree*, which is a way of presenting information about a choice. A decision tree visually links a decision maker's choices with the outcomes that are likely to result. It is called a tree because the possible outcomes branch from a choice. For the analyst, much of the value lies in the process of constructing the decision tree, as it highlights his or her perception of what will happen and where the information is weakest. In addition, many people find that examining a decision tree helps them understand the issues involved, as it lays out their best estimates of the cost or payoff and the probability associated with each possible outcome. As you can see in Figure 4.1, the worst-case forecast is a profit of $20,000, which is less than ideal, but not a catastrophe. Similarly, the best-case forecast is a profit of $120,000, which is good, but not superb. As is usually the case, laying out the decision tree helps clarify the

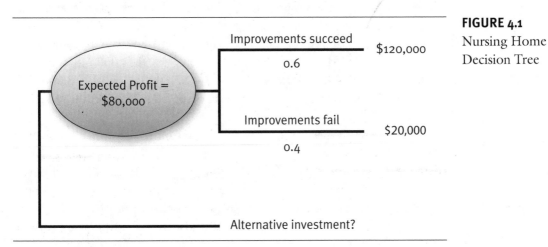

FIGURE 4.1

Nursing Home Decision Tree

situation by making the probability and profit estimates explicit. It does not tell managers what decision to make. As of yet, alternatives have not been laid out, so a sensible decision cannot be made.

Calculating the expected values of alternatives is sometimes called *rolling back* a decision tree. Rolling back a decision tree means calculating its expected value. In Figure 4.1, the expected return is $80,000.

Decision trees probably don't need to be drawn for scenarios as simple as this example, but a little more complexity can make construction of a tree worthwhile (see Figure 4.2). The consultant might well have noted that there is one chance in four that the state will reduce nursing home payments. If payments are reduced, profits will be $100,000 if the improvements succeed or $0 if they fail. The chance of rate cuts reduces expected profits to $75,000. The updated decision tree also displays the profit available from an alternative investment, in this case a short-term bond that returns $40,000. Most profit-oriented decision makers would prefer to invest in the nursing home, because its expected profit is higher and its outcomes with low profits do not entail losses.

Estimates of the variability of outcomes can be useful for making comparisons. Variability is typically measured by listing the range of possible values or by listing the *standard deviation* (which is the square root of the *variance*). If you are not comparing outcomes, the standard deviation is not helpful. In contrast, the range can convey useful information even if you are not comparing outcomes. The range helps you see the best- and worst-case scenarios. To know whether a risk is worth taking, you need to know the size of the risk and the potential payoff. Few people will want to take a risk if the best possible payoff is small or if the worst payoff is disastrous. On the other hand, if the best payoff is large, some people will be willing to accept significant risks.

To calculate variance, multiply the squared difference between the value of each outcome and the expected value by its probability of occurrence and then add the resulting products. (Note: you find the appropriate probability of occurrence by multiplying the probability on the "branch" of the outcome by the probability on the preceding branch.) So, in our example, the variance = $0.15 \times (\$100,000 - \$75,000)^2 + 0.45 \times (\$120,000 - \$75,000)^2 + 0.10 \times (\$0 - \$75,000)^2 + 0.3 \times (\$20,000 - \$75,000)^2$, or $2,475,000,000. The standard deviation is the square root of $2,475,000,000, which is $49,749.

A standard deviation or variance has meaning only when comparing options. If two choices have similar expected values, the one with the higher standard deviation carries a higher risk, as a larger standard deviation means that the bad outcomes are either more likely or much worse. For example, a project that has an 85 percent chance of earning $0 and a 15 percent chance of earning $500,000 also has an expected profit of

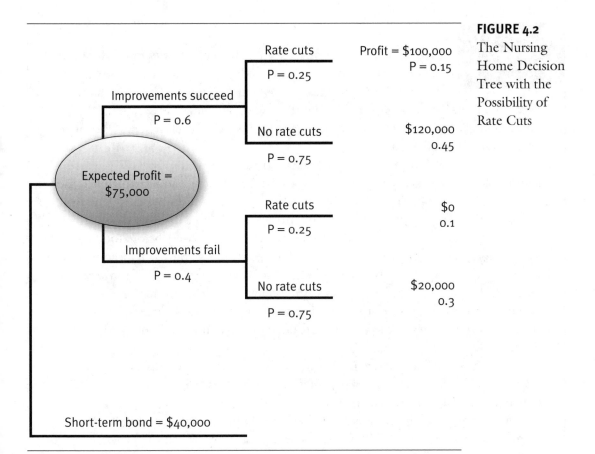

FIGURE 4.2

The Nursing Home Decision Tree with the Possibility of Rate Cuts

$75,000. The standard deviation for this project is $178,536, confirming its higher risk.

Remember, though, the point of these calculations is to improve your analysis. It should include an understanding of the size of the risk, how likely it is to occur, and whether it is worth taking. If your target audience, which might include members of the board or nonfinancial managers, is puzzled by your analysis and does not really understand the issues, you have failed to present it effectively. Your audience will not be able to offer useful feedback, and the decision to take or not take the risk will be all yours. Managers *could* be terminated for taking risks that the board and other managers understood and approved. Managers *will* be terminated for taking risks that the board and other managers did not understand.

4.3.1 Risk Preferences

Risk preferences may influence choices. A risk-seeking person prefers more variability. Someone who gambles in a casino must be a risk seeker because the expected payoff from a dollar bet will always be less than a dollar because of taxes and the casino's take. Likewise, a patient who can expect to

Case 4.2   **Investing in Cardiology Services at Western Regional Hospital**

"It's time for us to commit to building a center of excellence in cardiac care," said Shea Daniels, Western Regional Hospital's chief financial officer. "Mercy and Central did it three years ago, and they are doing extremely well. Medicare pays well, and the private insurers pay even better. We cannot afford to miss this opportunity."

"Perhaps," said Emerson Bruce, the hospital's chief medical officer. "Let me lay out a couple of issues that we need to consider. First, there's no guarantee that the insurers will keep on paying so well for cardiology services. Most observers think that prices are higher than they need to be, and Medicare is facing a financial crisis. I think that Medicare will move to a case rate for many cardiology services before too long. The cardiologists will continue to do nicely, but they will have powerful incentives to cut back on imaging, to cut back on catheterizations, and to switch to less invasive interventions. The net effect will be to slash hospital revenues. Second, there's no guarantee that we will be able to attract a team of top-notch cardiologists. Those guys are in short supply these days. Without a really superb team, we will not get this off the ground."

"OK," said Shea. "Here is what the planning team has forecast. We will need a 24-bed unit, office space for three cardiologists, a 64-slice CT scanner, and a cardiac catheterization lab. We estimate that this will cost us $10 million. We estimate that this will increase inpatient days by 1,500, resulting in profits of $2 million. We also estimate that we will have 1,000 new outpatient procedures, which will generate $500,000 in profits. That represents a very nice return on our investment and leaves us some room for error in our cost and revenue forecasts. Personally, I do not think that Medicare will make any changes fast. The ability of the federal government to avoid taking action is unsurpassed. And I am confident that we will be able to recruit cardiologists."

Discussion questions:
- How likely is a change in Medicare payment? What probability should you assign to it?
- What will happen to profits if Medicare does change its payment system?
- How likely is a failure to recruit three excellent cardiologists? What probability should you assign to this endeavor? What will happen to profits if you are able to recruit only two excellent cardiologists? If you set up this scenario as a decision tree, which of your assumptions become clear to other decision makers?
- What are the advantages of making your assumptions clear? What are the disadvantages?

live 18 months if he undergoes standard therapy may be a risk seeker. He may prefer a therapy that gives him an expected life span of only 13 months if it increases his chances of significant recovery. The manager of a nearly bankrupt business is likely also a risk seeker. Taking chances, even chances with low expected payoffs, may be the only way to survive.

A risk-neutral person does not care about variability and will always choose the outcome with the highest expected value. Large organizations with substantial reserves can afford to be risk neutral. For example, a firm with $400 million in cash reserves will probably not buy fire insurance for a $200,000 clinic. If the expected loss is $4,000 per year (a 2 percent chance of a $200,000 loss), the organization's fire insurance will cost at least $4,400 because of processing costs and insurer profits. On average, the firm will have higher profits if it does not insure this risk, and it can afford not to. Spending $200,000 for a new clinic will not put much of a dent in the organization's reserves.

A risk-averse person avoids variability and will sometimes choose strategies with smaller expected values to avoid risk. An individual who buys health insurance is likely to be risk averse, because the expected value of his or her covered expenses will usually be less than the premium. Insurance premiums must cover the insurer's expected payout, its cost of operation, and some return on invested capital. Unless a beneficiary's expected benefits (the insurer's expected payouts) have been incorrectly estimated, the insurer's costs and profits will push insurance premiums above expected losses. By definition, someone who will pay this is risk averse.

4.3.2 Decision Analysis

Formal decision analysis has three steps, and only one of them is difficult (Hammond, Keeney, and Raiffa 2002). The steps are setting up a decision tree; identifying the alternative with the largest expected value; and using sensitivity analysis to assess the robustness of the analysis. Setting up a decision tree is the hardest and most important part of decision analysis. Most insights are gained, but also most mistakes are made, in this step. Six steps are involved in setting up a decision tree.

1. Carefully define the problem. Often this task is harder than it sounds.
2. Identify the alternative courses of action. Serious mistakes are often made here.
3. Identify the outcomes associated with each alternative.
4. Identify the sequence of events leading to final outcomes. This sequence may include choices and chance events.
5. Calculate the probability of each outcome.
6. Calculate the value of each outcome.

Each of these steps is more difficult than it sounds, so often the first decision is whether to do a decision analysis at all.

4.3.3 Sensitivity Analysis

Any time setting up and solving a decision tree are worthwhile, performing a sensitivity analysis is equally worthwhile. A sensitivity analysis substitutes different, but plausible, values for the values in a decision tree. Gauging the effects of minor data changes on the results is always helpful. The data are never perfect, and using them as if they were would not make sense.

The decision tree for the nursing facility purchase tells us that the key issue is whether its manager can realize the operational improvements and product line changes that she is contemplating. If she can, the return on equity will be no less than 8.3 percent, no matter what Medicare does. A sensitivity analysis tells us that if she can realize about 70 percent of her projected gains, she can expect a 7 percent return on equity, no matter what Medicare does. What could she do to increase the odds of full improvement? The sensitivity analysis indicates that we can fall somewhat short of the manager's prediction and still hit the target rate of return.

4.4 Managing Risk

There are only two strategies for managing risk: risk sharing and diversification. Buying an insurance policy is the obvious way to share risk, although joint ventures or options can serve the same function. For insurance, consumers pay a fee to induce another organization to share risks; joint ventures or options share costs and profits with partners. Diversification can take a number of forms. Horizontal integration (creating an organization that can offer the full spectrum of healthcare services) is one diversification strategy, as some aspects of healthcare are likely to be profitable no matter what the environment. All of these strategies limit potential losses, but they also limit potential profitability.

Joint ventures and options are common in the biotechnology and pharmaceutical fields. For example, in 2008, StemCyte of Arcadia, California, announced the formation of a joint venture in India with Apollo Hospitals and Cadila Pharmaceuticals. The joint venture will provide stem cell therapies derived from umbilical cord blood to treat patients with leukemia, lymphoma, sickle cell anemia, and immune deficiency diseases. The joint venture will also provide a mechanism for the three companies to take part in clinical studies to develop new therapies. In a more mundane deal, in 2006 Ranbaxy Laboratories Limited announced a joint venture between it and Nippon Chemiphar

Limited of Japan. The joint venture will manufacture generic versions of Clarithromycin (an antibiotic) and Terbinafine (an antifungal), projecting Japanese sales of around $700 million. The products will be sold in Japan under the label of the joint venture and will be marketed jointly by the sales forces of the two parent companies. In a very different type of joint venture, Pfizer is joining Microsoft and IBM to create a system to automate physicians' offices. The need for automation is obvious to most observers, but none of the partners by itself had the skills and resources to develop and sell such a system to thousands of physicians.

These sorts of risk-sharing arrangements are not limited to the pharmaceutical industry or for-profit firms. The Sisters of Mercy sought to reorient their system from serving the suburbs to serving the inner-city poor. To do so, Mercy Health System built a new hospital in a blighted area. This initiative, however, created three problems: a massive bill for debt service, large losses on the new facility, and a lack of managers with experience serving this population. Mercy Health System addressed all three of these problems by entering into a joint venture with Henry Ford Health System. In exchange for an interest in two of Mercy's suburban facilities, Henry Ford offered protection against up to $4 million in annual losses on Mercy's new hospital and a CEO with experience serving the inner-city poor. This joint venture helped Mercy Health System better realize its goal, even though it was not profit driven (Flower 1993).

This example illustrates another facet of risk sharing. Often the cost that an organization seeks to share is the enormous cost of acquiring a key competency. Working with a knowledgeable partner allows the organization to gain experience. A lot of time and money is needed to build expertise, and joint ventures can reduce the risk of expending these resources needlessly. Of course the organization must also assess what the gains are for the partner, such as expertise and profits.

4.4.1 Diversification

Diversification consists of identifying a portfolio of projects or therapies that are not highly positively correlated. Table 4.1 compares investing in a clinic, investing in a trauma unit, and investing in a portfolio of 50 percent shares of each. Return on investment forecasts for the projects depend on whether the growth of an HMO is rapid, moderate, or slow. The clinic is a better investment than the trauma unit (higher expected profits and lower standard deviation of profits). The portfolio is also a better investment than the trauma unit (higher expected profits and lower standard deviation of profits). The portfolio might be a better investment than the clinic for a risk-averse investor (lower expected profits but a lower standard deviation of profits).

Case 4.3	**Diversification by Joint Venture**

The University of Pittsburgh Medical Center (UPMC) is partnering with the Beacon Medical Group to operate a hospital in Dublin, Ireland (UPMC 2008). UPMC already operates a transplant center in Italy, two cancer centers in Ireland, and a partnership to provide emergency care in Qatar. UPMC will pay about $22 million for a 25 percent stake in the operating company that will lease and operate Beacon Hospital. In addition, UPMC and Beacon are negotiating with the Irish government to operate three more hospitals that Beacon will build on the grounds of public hospitals. The joint venture with Beacon reduces the size of UPMC's investment and gives it a partner with local experience.

UPMC is headquartered in Pittsburgh, where it has a commanding presence. The largest employer in western Pennsylvania, with 48,000 employees and nearly $7 billion in revenue, UPMC owns 20 hospitals, 400 outpatient sites, a large insurance plan, and a number of other healthcare ventures. UPMC employs about half of the 5,000 physicians affiliated with it.

Despite its strong position, UPMC remains vulnerable to the performance of the local economy. Between 2001 and 2006, Pittsburgh lost 1.5 percent of its jobs, and the region lost 2.5 percent of its population. Much of UPMC's growth has resulted from acquisition of existing practice organizations, but its dominant position is likely to limit growth in the future. In addition, an ongoing concern is its relationship with Highmark BlueCross BlueShield, the dominant insurer in western Pennsylvania. And, like most healthcare organizations, UPMC remains vulnerable to changes in Medicare policies.

Discussion questions:
- Why is expansion outside the United States an attractive form of diversification?
- What are the pitfalls of international expansion?
- What are the potential pitfalls of other diversification efforts?
- Why is dependence on a small number of insurance plans a risk?
- Why is the slow growth of UPMC's home market a risk?

Joint ventures can make diversification less risky, as illustrated in Case 4.3.

4.5 Conclusion

The goal of describing, evaluating, and managing risk is improving choices, not identifying perfect choices. Even when the evidence available to a decision maker is good and he or she makes a good decision, bad outcomes can result. More often, though, medical and managerial decisions

	HMO Growth				Standard
	Rapid	Moderate	Slow	Expected	Deviation
Growth probabilities	0.160	0.700	0.140		
	Profits				
Clinic profits	10.0%	4.0%	−1.0%	4.3%	3.0%
Trauma unit profits	−3.0%	2.0%	13.0%	2.7%	4.5%
Portfolio profits (50% of each)	3.5%	3.0%	6.0%	3.5%	1.0%

TABLE 4.1
Diversification and Risk Reduction

are made with inadequate information. For example, managers often must make investment decisions long before they know how well technology will work, what volumes will be, and what rivals will do. Even when a manager has access to good information (which will never be the case with innovative choices), the possible consequences of his or her choices remain uncertain.

Good management, however, can reduce risk and reduce the consequences of risk. Some risks need not be taken because the payoff would not be adequate. Some risks can be shared via joint ventures or insurance. Some risks can be hedged via diversification. A balanced portfolio of projects and lines of business can be profitable in any market environment. Reducing variations in costs (so that risks are lower in capitated environments) or reducing fixed costs (so that sales slumps have fewer negative effects) can cut risk sharply. Finally, there's nothing like a high margin to reduce risk. If possible outcomes are a 15 percent return on equity or an 11 percent return on equity, most managers will sleep well.

Homework

4.1   Five of ten people earn $0, four earn $100, and one loses $100. What is the expected payoff? What is the variance of the payoff?

4.2   There is a 50 percent chance of making $0, a 40 percent chance of making $100, and a 10 percent chance of losing $100. Calculate the expected value and variance of the payoff. How does your estimate compare to the previous problem?

4.3   There is a 1 percent chance that you will have healthcare bills of
$100,000; a 19 percent chance that you will have healthcare bills of
$10,000; a 60 percent chance that you will have healthcare bills of
$500; and a 20 percent chance that you will have healthcare bills of
$0. What is your expected healthcare spending?

4.4   There is a 1 percent chance that you will have healthcare bills of
$100,000; a 19 percent chance that you will have healthcare bills of
$10,000; a 60 percent chance that you will have healthcare bills of
$500; and a 20 percent chance that you will have healthcare bills of
$0. What will your expected insurance benefits be? Would you be
willing to buy complete insurance coverage if it cost $3,712? Explain.

4.5   Instead of complete insurance, you have a policy with a $5,000
deductible. What will your expected out-of-pocket spending be? What
will your expected insurance benefits be? Assuming that the premium
equals 116 percent of expected insurance benefits, do you prefer the
policy with a $5,000 deductible or complete coverage? Explain.

4.6   Your firm, which operates a nationwide system of cancer clinics, has
annual profits of $800 million and cash reserves of $500 million. Your
clinics have a replacement value of $200 million, and fire insurance
for them would cost $5 million per year. Actuarial data show that
your expected losses due to fire are $4 million. Should you buy
insurance?

4.7   Your firm rents a supply management system to hospitals. You have
received a buyout offer of $5 million. You forecast that there is a
25 percent chance that you will have profits of $10 million, a
35 percent chance that you will have profits of $6 million, and a
40 percent chance that you will have profits of $2 million. Should you
accept the offer? Explain.

4.8   You were given a lottery ticket. The drawing will be held in 5 minutes.
You have a 0.1 percent chance of winning $10,000. You refuse an
offer of $11 for your ticket. Are you risk averse? Explain.

4.9   Your house is worth $200,000. Your risk of a catastrophic flood is
0.5 percent. Such a flood would destroy your house and would not be
covered by homeowner's insurance. Although you grumble, you buy
flood coverage for $1,200. Are you risk averse or risk seeking?

4.10 Your firm faces considerable revenue uncertainty because you have to
negotiate contracts with several customers. You forecast that there is a
20 percent chance that your revenues will be $200,000, a 30 percent
chance that your revenues will be $300,000, and a 50 percent chance
that your revenues will be $500,000. Your costs are also uncertain, as
the prices of your supplies fluctuate considerably. You forecast that

there is a 40 percent chance that your costs will be $400,000 and a 60 percent chance your costs will be $250,000. Use Excel to set up a decision tree for your profit forecast (it does not matter whether costs or revenues come first). How many possible profit outcomes do you have? What is your expected profit?

4.11 Your firm has been sued for $3 million by a supplier for breach of contract. Your lawyers believe that there are three possible outcomes if the suit goes to trial. One, which the lawyers term "highly improbable," is that your supplier will win the lawsuit and be awarded $3 million. Another, which the lawyers term "unlikely," is that your supplier will win the lawsuit and be awarded $500,000. The third, which the lawyers term "likely," is that your supplier will lose the lawsuit and be awarded $0. You have to decide whether to try to settle the case. To do so you need to assign probabilities to "highly improbable," "unlikely," and "likely." What probabilities correspond to these statements? Going to trial will cost you $100,000 in legal fees. One of your lawyers believes that your supplier will settle for $100,000 (and you will have legal fees of $25,000). Should you settle?

Chapter Glossary

Decision tree. A visual decision support tool that depicts the values and probabilities of the outcomes of a choice

Expected value. The sum of the probability of each possible outcome multiplied by the value of the outcome

Objective probability. An estimate of probability based on observed frequencies

Range. The difference between the largest and smallest values of a variable

Risk aversion. The reluctance of a decision maker to accept an outcome with an uncertain payoff rather than a smaller, more certain outcome (A risk-averse person would prefer getting $5 for sure to a gamble with a 50 percent chance of getting nothing and a 50 percent chance of getting $10.)

Risk neutrality. The indifference of a decision maker to risk (A risk-neutral person would think that getting $5 for sure is as good as a gamble with a 50 percent chance of getting nothing and a 50 percent chance of getting $10.)

Risk seeking. The preference of a decision maker for risk (A risk-seeking person would prefer a gamble with a 50 percent chance of getting nothing and a 50 percent chance of getting $10 to getting $5 for sure.)

Sensitivity analysis. The process of varying the assumptions in an analysis over a reasonable range and observing how the outcome changes

Standard deviation. The square root of a variance

Subjective probability. An individual's judgment about how likely a particular event is to occur

Variance. The squared deviation of a random variable from its expected value (If a variable takes the value 3 with a probability of 0.2, the value 6 with a probability of 0.3, and the value 9 with a probability of 0.5, its expected value is 6.9. Its variance is 5.49, which is $0.2 \times [3 - 6.9]^2 + 0.3 \times [6 - 6.9]^2 + 0.5 \times [9 - 6.9]^2$.)

References

Congressional Budget Office. 2007. "Medicare Advantage: Private Health Plans in Medicare." [Online information; retrieved 3/14/08.] www.cbo.gov/ftpdocs/82xx/doc8268/06-28-Medicare_Advantage.pdf.

Flower, J. 1993. "Catalyzing the Community." [Online information; retrieved 12/6/08.] www.well.com/~bbear/catalyze.html.

Hammond, J. S., R. L. Keeney, and H. Raiffa. 2002. *Smart Choices: A Practical Guide to Making Better Decisions.* New York: Broadway.

University of Pittsburgh Medical Center (UPMC). 2008. "UPMC to Manage Independent Hospital in Dublin, Ireland." [Online information; retrieved 1/12/09.] www.upmc.com/MediaRelations/NewsReleases/2008/Pages/Ireland-BMG.aspx.

UNDERSTANDING COSTS

After reading this chapter, students will be able to:

- **calculate** average and marginal costs,
- **articulate** why efficiency is important,
- **identify** opportunity costs,
- **forecast** how changes in technology and prices will change costs, and
- **discuss** the relationship between cost and quality.

Key Concepts

- Costs depend on perspective.
- Costs can be hard to measure.
- Good managers have an accurate understanding of costs.
- Goods and services an organization produces are called *outputs*.
- Goods and services an organization uses in production are called *inputs*.
- *Incremental cost* equals the change in cost resulting from a change in output.
- *Average cost* equals the total cost of a process divided by the total output of a process.
- Large firms have a cost advantage if there are *economies of scale*.
- Multiproduct firms have a cost advantage if there are *economies of scope*.
- Higher quality should mean higher costs. If not, the organization is inefficient.
- Higher input prices mean higher costs.
- Costs depend on outputs, technology, input prices, and efficiency.
- *Opportunity cost* is the value of a resource in its best alternative use.
- *Sunk costs*, which are costs you cannot change, should be ignored.

5.1 Understanding Costs

Understanding and managing costs are core managerial tasks. Whatever the mission of the organization, cost control must be a priority. As evidence

Case 5.1   **Virginia Mason Medical Center**

In 2001, Virginia Mason Medical Center was under pressure to improve its financial performance. Its processes of care were overrun with waste and rework, increasing costs and putting patients at risk (Nelson-Peterson and Leppa 2007).

Virginia Mason used week-long rapid process improvement workshops to examine processes, measure wasted resources, and identify activities that did not add value for customers. Workshop participants included leaders and frontline staff, supported by executive sponsors and performance improvement experts. After identifying areas for improvement, workshop participants discussed ways to standardize and optimize the work that would need to be done. Preliminary data collection (including observations of how care was delivered) started weeks before the workshops, and follow-up continued for months.

In 2005, an eight-person team (including a patient) participated in a workshop focused on a 27-bed telemetry unit that was experiencing numerous problems. Nurses were assigned patients with no consideration of how sick the patients were or where they were located, resulting in varied workloads and unnecessary travel between rooms. Supplies and equipment were not kept where they were needed. The work of nurses and technicians was poorly coordinated; some things were done twice, and some things were not done at all. Communication was poor, patient status changes were missed too often, and nurses felt pressured to skip breaks and lunches. Furthermore, the unit's financial performance was unsatisfactory because it was consistently staffing over budget.

The workshop team made a number of simple changes that dramatically streamlined care. First, they changed staff assignments so that nurses cared for patients in contiguous rooms, reducing travel by 85 percent. Second, they moved supplies to

mounts that many healthcare firms are inefficient, cost control in the healthcare industry is becoming increasingly important. A firm is inefficient when its costs are higher than the quality of its service warrants, when the quality of a firm's products is lower than the cost of its service warrants, or when the quality of a firm's products is lower and its costs are higher than the quality and costs of comparable competitors.

An efficient producer of a good or service has a competitive advantage. For example, a pharmacy that can accurately dispense a product more cheaply than its competitors has an advantage. The efficient producer can win more contracts, enjoy higher profit margins, or more easily weather a slump. In healthcare, the bar has been raised, as increased attention to the outcomes of care challenges us to think about health, not just medical care. Healthcare organizations are being challenged to work with cus-

where they were needed and simplified ordering, reducing the time spent retrieving supplies by 85 percent. Third, they standardized and streamlined morning rounds, shortening them by 48 percent. As a result of these changes, costs and overtime hours dropped, patient falls and pressure ulcers decreased, patient satisfaction improved, and call light use fell.

Nonetheless, the nurses' initial response to these changes was not positive. They wanted to focus on caring for patients rather than on improving financial performance. In addition, they were not happy with the standardization of their work and resisted some of the proposed changes. Managers had to be present on the unit every day for a number of weeks to ensure that the nurses followed the new strategy.

Over the next several months, the nurses' response became more positive. They could see that care had improved and that they were not as exhausted at the end of their shifts. Skipping breaks and meals ceased to be routine practice. In informal comments and in surveys, the nurses expressed higher levels of satisfaction.

Discussion questions:

- Did standardizing care reduce quality? Did standardizing care reduce costs? What evidence supports your conclusions?
- How would reducing travel time between rooms reduce costs?
- Does including a patient in the rapid process improvement workshop make sense? Why?
- Was Virginia Mason efficient before it made these changes? Who is responsible for ensuring that care is efficient?
- Why did the nurses resist the changes? Would you expect to encounter resistance in other departments?

tomers to produce health efficiently, not just to produce goods and services efficiently.

This chapter focuses on what is necessary to turn an organization into an efficient producer. The starting point is to understand costs, which are defined by a combination of two definitions. First, the goods or services an organization uses in producing its outputs are called *inputs*. Second, *opportunity cost* equals the value of an input in its best alternative use. From this production-oriented perspective, costs equal the opportunity cost per unit of input multiplied by the volume of inputs the organization uses. Reducing the cost per unit that the organization pays for inputs reduces total costs, but real savings result from reducing the volume of inputs the organization uses. To reduce input volume, managers must lead efficiency improvement efforts or outsource the production of goods and services.

5.2 Cost Perspectives

Cost is a complex concept because it is difficult to measure and depends on the perspective of the beholder. For example, consumers will characterize the cost of a prescription in terms of their out-of-pocket spending and ancillary costs, such as the value of time spent filling a prescription. Pharmacists will focus on the spending required to obtain, store, and dispense the drug. Insurers will focus on their payments to the pharmacist for the prescription and their spending on claim management. Each of these perspectives on costs is valid. Table 5.1 describes what costs look like from four perspectives.

A pharmacist acquires a prescription drug for $10 and incurs $5 in processing, storing, and billing costs. The pharmacist should recognize that a reasonable return on her time and on her investment in the pharmacy represents opportunity costs, as both could be used in other ways.

The consumer is uninterested in the pharmacist's costs. What matters to him are his out-of-pocket costs and the $4 in travel expense he incurs when he drives to the pharmacy. When the consumer does not have insurance, as shown in the left half of Table 5.1, the consumer's perspective on costs mirrors society's perspective. Both will say that the drug costs $20, although the two calculations are different. The consumer will focus on the price he pays and his travel costs. Society will ignore the price the consumer pays and focus on the underlying resource use by the pharmacist and the consumer. The payment is an accounting entry, not a real use of resources (because it equals the amount the pharmacist receives).

The right side of Table 5.1 lists cost perspectives when the prescription is covered by insurance. Three things change as a result of coverage.

TABLE 5.1
Costs from
Four
Perspectives

	Cost of a Prescription Without Insurance			Cost of a Prescription with Insurance			
	Pharmacy	*Consumer*	*Society*	*Pharmacy*	*Consumer*	*Insurer*	*Society*
Wholesale price	$10	$0	$10	$10	$0	$0	$10
Travel	$0	$4	$4	$0	$4	$0	$4
Processing	$5	$0	$5	$5	$0	$9	$14
Return on assets	$1	$0	$1	$1	$0	$1	$2
Retail price	($16)	$16	$0	($16)	$5	$11	$0
Total	$0	$20	$20	$0	$9	$21	$30

First, there is an additional perspective to consider, that of the insurer. Second, the insurer incurs expense by processing the claim. Third, the consumer's perspective on costs differs from society's perspective.

The insurer focuses on its share of the retail price and its cost of paying the bill. Again, the insurer should factor in the opportunity cost of using its investment to provide pharmacy insurance benefits but will probably express this figure in terms of a required return on investment. From the perspective of the insurer, covering the prescription adds $21 in costs. From the perspective of the consumer, insurance coverage reduces costs by $11. Note also that society's perspective on costs differs from the perspective of any of the participants when insurance plays a role.

If you do not state a cost perspective, you do not fully understand the concept of cost. The part of costs that matters depends on your point of view. Your revenues are someone else's costs, and your costs are someone else's revenues.

Most people want to focus on costs from the perspective of the organization in which they work, but shifting costs to customers or suppliers seldom represents a good business strategy. Long-term business success rests on selling products that offer your customers excellent value and offer your suppliers adequate profits.

As stated earlier, the difficulty of measuring cost components also complicates the concept of costs. For example, opportunity costs are sometimes hard to measure. Managers sometimes become confused when calculating the opportunity cost of resources that have changed in value. For example, land that your organization bought a few years ago may be more valuable if rents in the area have risen or less valuable if rents have fallen. In most cases, though, an input's opportunity cost is simply its market price.

Linking the use of a resource to the organization's output also poses problems. A focus on incremental costs (i.e., the cost of the additional resources you use when you increase output by a small amount) often simplifies this task. "How much more of a hospital's information system does its intensive care unit use when it cares for an additional patient?" is an example of a way to reframe the relationship between resource use and output and facilitate its measurement.

5.3 Vocabulary

To talk sensibly about costs, we need a clear vocabulary. At the core of that vocabulary are the concepts of average cost and incremental cost. *Average cost* equals the total cost of a process divided by the total output of a process. In Table 5.2, when total cost equals $10,500 and output equals

300, average cost equals $35. *Incremental cost*, also called *marginal cost*, equals the change in a process's total cost that is associated with a change in the process's total output. In Table 5.2, total cost rises from $8,000 to $10,500 as output rises from 200 to 300, so incremental cost equals ($10,500 − $8,000) ÷ (300 − 200), or $25 per unit of output.

In Table 5.2, average cost is significantly larger than incremental cost. This difference is common because many processes require resources (such as equipment or key personnel) that do not change as output varies. For example, to open a pharmacy, a pharmacist has to rent a building and commit her own time. If sales fall short of expectations, the rent will not change. Rent is an example of a *fixed cost*, a component of total cost. In contrast, some labor costs and the cost of restocking the pharmacy will vary with sales. Average cost includes fixed and variable costs, but incremental cost includes only variable costs. The fact that average cost often exceeds incremental cost is important because management decisions often hinge on knowing how much increasing or decreasing production of a good or service will cost. Your willingness to negotiate with an insurer that offers $300 per service is likely to depend on whether you believe an additional service will cost you $440 (the average cost) or $120 (the incremental cost).

Average and incremental cost are both important concepts, although economists emphasize incremental values. Most management decisions concern incremental changes. Should we increase hours in the pediatric clinic? Should we reduce evening pharmacy staff? Should we accept patients needing skilled nursing care? These sorts of decisions demand data on incremental costs.

In addition to being the most relevant concept for managers, incremental cost is easier to calculate than average cost. Average cost calculations always involve difficult questions (e.g., How much of the cost incurred by the chief financial officer should we allocate to the pediatrics department?). In contrast, incremental cost calculations involve more straightforward questions and can be performed by most clinicians and frontline managers (e.g., What additional resources will we need to keep the pediatric clinic open until 8 p.m. on Wednesdays, and what are the opportunity costs of those

TABLE 5.2

Total, Average, and Incremental Costs

Output	Total Cost	Average Cost	Incremental Cost
0	$3,000		
100	$5,500	$55	$25
200	$8,000	$40	$25
300	$10,500	$10,500/300 = $35	$2,500/100 = $25

resources?). To decide whether to start or stop a service, a manager needs to compare average revenue and average cost. For example, a telemedicine program that has average revenue of $84 and average cost of $98 is unprofitable. To decide whether to expand or contract a service, a manager needs to compare how revenue and costs will change. To make this comparison, information about incremental costs is essential. Usually confusion about cost arises because one person is talking about average cost and another is talking about incremental cost (or because one person is talking about costs to society and the other is talking about costs to the organization).

5.4 Factors That Influence Costs

Producer costs depend on what is produced (the outputs), the prices of inputs, how outputs are produced (the technology), and how efficiently inputs are used. We will explore each of these factors.

5.4.1 Outputs

Differences in outputs can profoundly affect costs. Firms that produce large volumes of a good or service may have lower costs than firms that produce small volumes. Large firms that have a cost advantage have *economies of scale*. Firms that produce several different kinds of goods or services may have lower costs than firms that produce just one. Multiproduct firms that have a cost advantage have *economies of scope*. Economies of scale and scope result from sharing resources.

An example of economies of scale might be a large pharmacy's use of automated dispensing equipment. In a larger pharmacy the fixed costs of the equipment could be shared by a larger number of prescriptions, so the cost per prescription could be lower. An example of economies of scope might be a nursing home that expanded to offer skilled care as well as intermediate care. Fixed costs (such as the cost of the director of nursing) would now be shared by additional patients, so average costs for intermediate care could be lower.

Differences in the quality of outputs can affect costs as well. For an efficient firm, higher-quality products cost more. For an inefficient firm, higher-quality products may not.

What is higher quality? Economists define *quality* from the perspective of consumers, not from the clinical perspective common in healthcare. In economics, a good or service is of higher quality when it is more valuable to a well-informed customer than comparable goods or services. Consumers usually find greater value in goods or services that produce better clinical outcomes. Economists also define quality in terms of nonclinical factors. Well-informed consumers may attribute higher quality to a product that is

Case 5.2   **Improving Performance**

"It's just another management fad. This Six Sigma stuff will fade into the mists of time. Remember Management by Walking Around? When was the last time anyone talked about that?" said Tyler Austin, chief medical officer of Westview Hospital, on a rant.

"Perhaps," said Jordan Williams, director of performance improvement, "but the basic ideas are hard to argue with. Figure out what you want to do, figure out what you are actually doing, try some new ways of doing things, choose some combination of improvements as your new standard practice, then track performance to make sure it has gotten better and is staying that way. Its terminology—define, measure, analyze, improve, and control—may not last, but the ideas are hardly trendy.

"Take a look at what Virtua Home Care accomplished (Elberfeld et al. 2007). After Medicare switched from cost-based reimbursement to case-based reimbursement in 2000, Virtua was in a lot of trouble. It was losing money, volume was down, and poor quality was resulting in deficiencies. Its choices were to change or close. In conjunction with the leadership of the system, its executive director chose to change. Focusing on 2 of its 12 clinical teams, Virtua brought together the directors of nursing, improvement experts, and a number of frontline staff. After a detailed analysis, the team concluded that Virtua was doing a poor job of documenting care and was not delivering the care it was supposed to. The documentation problems included high documentation costs, late bills, large numbers of defective bills, and large numbers of denials. The care delivery problems included referral failures and coordination failures. Both problems increased costs and reduced revenues.

easier to use, a service for which the wait is shorter, an insurance plan with less confusing referral requirements, a provider who bills more accurately, or a more cordial staff.

If higher quality does not cost more, failure to provide it demonstrates inefficiency. The many opportunities healthcare presently has to improve quality without increasing costs reflect how inefficient most healthcare organizations are. Once an organization has become efficient, though, higher quality (better service, improved reliability, greater accuracy, less pain, and other enhancements) will cost more to produce.

5.4.2 Input Costs

Higher input prices mean higher costs. Shifting to a different combination of inputs will only partially offset the effects of higher input prices. The only times this rule does not hold are when a firm is inefficient or when there is a perfect, lower-priced substitute for the higher-priced input. An inefficient firm

"To make a long story short," Jordan concluded, "Virtua simplified and standardized its billing, documentation, and referral processes. It also developed a set of simple reports so that everyone in the agency could track performance. The bottom line was that revenues went up, costs went down, and the clinical quality of care improved. Profits improved enough to allow Virtua to buy a new clinical information system that allowed it to further simplify and standardize operations. We need to do something like that. Don't call it Six Sigma if that bothers you, but we need to do something like that."

Discussion questions:
- Why did switching to a case rate from cost-based reimbursement put pressure on home health agencies?
- How could a bad job of documentation cost more than a good job?
- Why would poor documentation hurt revenue?
- Why would poor documentation hurt clinical quality?
- Some of your nurses are objecting to efforts to standardize care, calling it cookbook nursing. How do you respond?
- What would have happened to Virtua's employees if the agency had continued to lose money?
- Was Virtua efficient before it made the changes described in this case?
- Are Virtua's problems with documentation, communication, and coordination unusual? Do other healthcare firms have similar problems? How do such problems affect profits and clinical quality?

might be able to limit the effects of a cost increase by shifting to a more efficient production process. For example, even if the wages of pharmacy technicians increase, the cost of dispensing a prescription might not increase if the pharmacy switches to the automated system it should have been using before the wage increase. A firm also can avoid higher costs by switching to a perfect substitute. For example, if an Internet access provider tried to raise its monthly rates, firms could switch to rival Internet access providers and costs would not go up. Unfortunately, firms are unlikely to find such a replacement.

5.4.3 Technology
Advances in technology always reduce the cost of an activity. Adopting a new technology would be pointless if it increased the costs of a process. For example, installing an automated laboratory system would be absurd if it increased cost per analysis. An automated laboratory system that reduces cost per analysis, however, does not guarantee that laboratory costs will go down.

Lower costs per analysis may prompt physicians to request more analyses, and the greater volume cancels the cost savings and might even drive up costs.

5.4.4 Efficiency

Increases in efficiency always reduce the cost of an activity. Production of almost every healthcare good or service can be made more efficient. Few production processes in healthcare have been examined carefully, and most healthcare workers have little or no training in process improvement. Consequently, mistakes, delays, coordination failures, unwise input choices, and excess capacity are routine. Techniques for improving production (total quality management, continuous quality improvement, and continuous process improvement) are just beginning to be applied in healthcare, so there is much to be done.

Even though greater efficiency reduces costs, not everyone is in favor of it. Greater efficiency often means that fewer workers will be needed. Workers whose jobs are in jeopardy may not want to help improve efficiency. (Commitment to a policy of no layoffs is usually one of the core terms of efficiency improvements.) Others have limited incentive to participate in efforts to improve efficiency. Physicians must help change clinical processes, yet many physicians have little to gain from these efforts. The gains produced by the changes will accrue to the healthcare organization, but the resulting billing reductions will be problematic for physicians and other healthcare workers not employed by the organization. A major challenge lies in devising incentives that will encourage workers and contractors to help improve efficiency.

5.5 Variable and Fixed Costs

An understanding of opportunity costs and triggers that change costs is required to manage costs. As stated earlier, opportunity costs usually are easy to assess. The opportunity cost of using $220 in supplies is $220. The opportunity cost of using an hour of legal time billed at $150 per hour is $150. Other cases demand more study. For example, the opportunity cost of a vacant wing of a hospital depends on its future use. If the wing will be reopened for acute care in response to a rising hospital census, the opportunity cost of the wing will depend on its value as an acute care unit. If the wing will be reopened because the hospital needs a skilled nursing unit, the opportunity cost of the wing will be determined by its value in that role.

Sunk costs should be ignored. A *sunk cost* is a cost you cannot change. A computer's purchase price is a sunk cost, as is money you spent to train employees to operate the computer. If your current needs do not require the use of a computer, you should not fret about its initial cost. The opportunity cost of the computer will depend on its value in some other use (including its resale value).

In the long run, all costs are variable. Buildings and equipment can be changed or built. The way work is done can be changed. Additional personnel can be hired. The entire organization could shut down, and its assets could be sold.

In the short run, some costs are fixed. An existing lease may not be negotiable, even if the building or equipment no longer suits your needs. Ignore fixed costs in the short run. They are sunk costs.

When there are substantial fixed costs, average costs typically fall as output increases because the fixed costs are being spread over a growing volume of output. As long as average variable costs are stable, this drop in average fixed costs will cause a reduction in average total costs. *Average total costs* equal average fixed costs plus average variable costs. As Table 5.3 illustrates, average fixed cost drops from $30 to $15 as output rises from 100 to 200. If variable costs rise quickly enough, average total costs may rise despite the fall in average fixed costs. In Table 5.3, variable costs rise by $10,000 as output increases from 200 to 300. As a result, average total cost rises to $60 even though average fixed cost continues to fall.

Fixed and variable costs are important concepts for day-to-day management of healthcare organizations. For example, an advantage of growth is that fixed costs can be spread over a larger volume of output. The idea is that lower average fixed costs result in lower average total costs, so profit margins can be larger. As Table 5.3 illustrates, growth should not result in increases in average variable costs large enough to offset any reduction in average fixed costs. Otherwise, growth will be unprofitable.

Misclassification of costs can result in odd incentives. For example, fixed overhead costs are often allocated on the basis of some measure of output, which can make growth appear less profitable than it is because the overhead costs allocated to a unit increase as it grows. So that unit managers are not discouraged from expanding, allocated fixed costs should not vary with output.

TABLE 5.3

Fixed and Variable Costs

Output	Total Cost	Fixed Cost	Average Total Cost	Average Fixed Cost	Average Variable Cost
0	$3,000	$3,000			
100	$5,500	$3,000	$55	$30	$25
200	$8,000	$3,000	$40	$15	$25
300	$18,000	$3,000	$18,000 /300 = $60	$3,000/300 = $10	$15,000/300 = $50

Case 5.3   **The Costs of Non-Urgent Care in the Emergency Department**

"Obviously," said Kelly Santo, director of patient accounts, Happy Hospital, "it costs more to see a patient in the emergency department than in a physician's office. We've got to channel these folks back to their primary care physicians. Plus, most of these folks don't have insurance, so they are money losers for us."

Emerson Campbell, director of emergency services, replied, "Actually, it's more complicated than that. Most patients seen in our emergency department have insurance, and it is not clear whether we are making money on them. There have been a couple of careful studies of costs in emergency departments, but they reach different conclusions. A study by R. M. Williams (1996) concluded that the incremental cost of a patient visit for routine ambulatory care was not high and that these patients were quite profitable for hospitals. A subsequent study by A. Bamezai, G. A. Melnick, and A. Nawathe in 2005 found much higher costs. Emergency departments produce such a range of services, and there is so much overhead to allocate, that figuring out how much it costs to care for a child with an earache at 2 a.m. is a nightmare. We'd be happy to do a detailed cost analysis of the emergency department, but we have had other priorities up to now."

At that point, Morgan McKenna, chief executive, chimed in, "Let's think strategically here. First, I'll bet a month's pay that we could reduce costs in the emergency department and improve the experience of our patients, critically ill or not. Doing so will increase profits, whatever our costs are. Second, our emergency department is overcrowded. We need to develop the capacity to see patients who are not critically ill more efficiently. Most of these patients do not need the sort of sophisticated care that our emergency department provides, and our emergency department was on diversion for eight days last month. That is not acceptable. Emerson, I want you and Kelly to develop a menu of options for our next meeting."

Discussion questions:
- Why do patients who are not critically ill go to emergency departments?
- Why do the variety of services emergency departments produce and the amount of overhead to be allocated make cost finding difficult?
- Why was Morgan McKenna confident that costs could be reduced while quality could be improved? Is this conclusion supported in the literature?
- Thinking as a consumer, what would constitute higher quality in emergency department services? What options should the hospital consider? Why would you be confident that they would incur lower costs than an emergency department? Do you think quality would be higher?

5.6 Conclusion

Cost management has become vital in healthcare. A more efficient producer always has an advantage. The increasingly competitive environment is forcing healthcare organizations to reduce costs and reassess product lines. More and more, healthcare organizations are seeking the cheapest production techniques and identifying core goods and services. This pressure has intensified as purchasers of goods and services have realized that high costs do not guarantee high quality and that high quality does not necessarily equate to high cost. Healthcare organizations are beginning to adopt cost-reducing technology, substitute high-cost for low-cost production techniques, purchase goods and services more conservatively, and rethink what they produce. Healthcare providers are also being challenged to improve the health of target populations in ways that are cost-effective—a task that is more difficult than the efficient production of healthcare products.

Homework

5.1   Why is it important to distinguish between fixed and variable costs?

5.2   Explain how a decrease in input prices or an increase in efficiency would affect costs.

5.3   You spent $500,000 on staff training last year. Why should this be treated as a sunk cost? Why should this cost be ignored in making a decision whether to switch coding software?

5.4   Your president bought two acres of land for $200,000 ten years ago. Although it is zoned for commercial use, it currently houses eight small, single-family houses. A property management firm that wants to continue leasing the eight houses has offered you $400,000 for the property. A developer wants to build a 12-story apartment building on the site and has offered $600,000. What value should you assign to the property?

5.5   A community health center has assembled the following data on cost and volume. Calculate its average and marginal costs for volumes ranging from 25 to 40. What patterns do you see?

Visits	Total Cost
20	$2,200
25	$2,250
30	$2,300
35	$2,350
40	$2,400

5.6   Sweetwater Nursing Home has 150 beds. Its cost and volume data are in the table below. Calculate its average and marginal costs for volumes ranging from 100 to 140. What patterns do you see?

Residents	Costs
80	$10,000
100	$11,000
120	$12,000
140	$13,200

5.7   It takes a phlebotomist 15 minutes to complete a blood draw. The supplies for each draw cost $4, and the phlebotomist earns $20 per hour. The phlebotomy lab is designed to accommodate 20,000 draws per year. Its rent is $80,000 per year. What are the average and incremental costs of a blood draw when the volume is 20,000? 10,000? What principle does your calculation illustrate?

5.8   How would the average and marginal costs change if the phlebotomist's wage rose to $24 per hour? What principle does your calculation illustrate?

5.9   A new computer lets a phlebotomist complete a blood draw in 10 minutes. The supplies for each draw cost $4, and the phlebotomist earns $20 per hour. The phlebotomy lab is designed to accommodate 20,000 draws per year. Its rent is $80,000 per year. What is the marginal cost of a blood draw? What principle does your calculation illustrate?

5.10 Use the data in question 5.7. How would the average and marginal costs change if the rent rose to $100,000? What principle does your calculation illustrate?

5.11 A patient visits a clinic. She incurs $10 in travel costs and has a copay of $20. The clinic's total charge is $60. The clinic spends $9 to bill the insurance company for the visit and uses resources worth $51 to produce the visit. The insurance company pays the clinic $40 and spends $11 to process the claim. Describe the cost of the visit from the perspective of the patient, the clinic, the insurer, and society.

5.12 A practice uses $40 worth of a dentist's time, $30 worth of a hygienist's time, $10 worth of supplies, and $15 worth of a billing clerk's time to produce a visit. The practice charges a patient $25 and charges her insurer $70. The insurer spends an additional $4 to process the claim. The patient incurs travel costs of $20. What are the costs of the visit from the perspective of society, the patient, the practice, and the insurer?

5.13 Kim and Pat underwrite insurance. Each underwrites 50 accounts per month. Each account takes four hours to underwrite. The value of their time is $40 per hour. Monthly costs for each are $1,500 for an office, $2,000 for a receptionist, and $2,400 for a secretary. Calculate the average and incremental cost per case for Kim and Pat.

5.14 If Kim and Pat merge their operations, they would need only one receptionist and their rent for the joint office would be $2,800 per month. All other values stay the same. Calculate the average and incremental cost per case for the merged office. Are there economies of scale at 100 accounts per month? Should Kim and Pat merge their offices?

Chapter Glossary

Average cost. Total cost divided by total output

Case-based payment. A single payment for an episode of care (The payment does not change if fewer services or more services are provided.)

Economies of scale. When larger organizations have lower average costs

Economies of scope. When multiproduct organizations have lower average costs

Efficient. Productive of the most valuable output possible, given its inputs (Viewed differently, an efficient organization uses the least expensive inputs possible, given the quality and quantity of output it produces.)

Factor of production. Another name for an input

Fixed costs. Costs that do not vary according to output

Input. A good or service used in the production of another good or service

Marginal analysis. Assessment of the effects of small changes in a decision variable (such as price or the volume of output) on outcomes (such as costs, profits, or the probability of recovery)

Marginal or incremental cost. The cost of producing an additional unit of output

Normal rate of return. A profit rate that is high enough to retain current factors of production in an industry or occupation and low enough not to attract new entrants (The normal rate of return will equal the opportunity cost of the factors.)

Opportunity cost. The value of a resource in its next best use (The opportunity cost of a product consists of the other goods and services we cannot have because we have chosen to produce the product in question.)

Output. The good or service that emerges from a production process

Sunk costs. Costs that have been incurred and cannot be recouped

References

Bamezai, A., G. A. Melnick, and A. Nawathe. 2005. "The Cost of an ED Visit and Its Relationship to ED Volume." *Annals of Emergency Medicine* 45 (5): 483–90.

Elberfeld, A., S. Benni, J. Ritzius, and D. Yhlen. 2007. "The Innovative Use of Six Sigma in Home Care." *Home Healthcare Nurse* 25 (1): 25–33.

Nelson-Peterson, D. L., and C. J. Leppa. 2007. "Creating an Environment for Caring Using Lean Principles of the Virginia Mason Production System." *Journal of Nursing Administration* 37 (6): 287–94.

Williams, R. M. 1996. "The Costs of Visits to Emergency Departments." *New England Journal of Medicine* 334 (10): 642–46.

THE DEMAND FOR HEALTHCARE PRODUCTS

Learning Objectives

After reading this chapter, students will be able to:

- **calculate** sales and revenue using simple models,
- **discuss** the importance of demand in management decision making,
- **articulate** why consumer demand is an important topic in healthcare,
- **apply** demand theory to anticipate the effects of a policy change,
- **use** standard terminology to describe the demand for healthcare products, and
- **discuss** the factors that influence demand.

Key Concepts

- The *quantity demanded* is the amount of a good or service purchased at a specific price when all other factors are held constant.
- When a product's price rises, the quantity demanded usually falls.
- *Demand* (a demand curve) describes the amounts of a good or service that will be purchased at different prices when all other factors are held constant.
- *Market demand* is the sum of the demands of all consumers in a market.
- An *increase or decrease in demand* reflects a shift in the entire list of amounts purchased at different prices. An increase or a decrease in demand results when another factor that influences consumer decisions changes.
- Other factors that influence demand include consumer income, insurance coverage, perceptions of health status, perceptions of the productivity of goods and services, prices of other goods and services, and tastes.
- The amount of money a consumer herself pays for a good or service is called the *out-of-pocket price* of that good or service.
- Because of insurance, the total price and the out-of-pocket price can differ quite a bit.

- A *complement* is a good or service that is used in conjunction with another good or service. Demand for a good falls if the price of a complement increases.
- A *substitute* is a good or service used instead of another good or service. Demand for a good rises if a substitute increases in price.

6.1 Introduction

Demand is one of the central ideas of economics. It underpins many of economics' contributions to public and private decision making. Analyses of demand tell us that human wants are seldom absolute. More often they are conditioned by questions: "Is it really worth it?" "Is its value greater than its cost?" These questions are central to understanding healthcare economics.

Demand forecasts are essential to management. Most managerial decisions are based on revenue projections. Revenue projections in turn depend on estimates of sales volume, given prices that managers set. A volume estimate is an application of demand theory. An understanding of the relationship between price and quantity must be part of every manager's tool kit. On an even more fundamental level, demand forecasts help managers decide whether to produce a certain product at all and how much to charge. Suppose you conclude that the direct costs of providing therapeutic massage are $48 and that you will need to charge at least $75 to cover other costs and offer an attractive profit margin. Will you have enough customers to make this a sensible addition to your product line? Demand analyses are designed to answer such questions.

On an abstract level, we need to ration goods and services (including medical goods and services) somehow. Human wants are infinite, or nearly so. Our capacity to satisfy those wants is finite. We must develop a system for determining which wants will be satisfied and which will not. Market systems use prices to ration goods and services. A price system costs relatively little to operate, is usually self-correcting (e.g., prices fall when the quantity supplied exceeds the quantity demanded, which tends to restore balance), and allows individuals with different wants to make different choices. These are important advantages. The problem is that markets work by limiting the choices of some consumers. As a result, even if the market *process* is fair, the market *outcome* may seem unfair. Wealthy societies typically view exclusion of some consumers from valuable medical services, perhaps because of low income or perhaps because of previous catastrophic medical expenses, as unacceptable.

The implications of demand are not limited to market-oriented systems, however. Demand theory predicts that if care is not rationed by

---

Sidebar 6.1 Using Demand Forecasts

Longs Drug Stores uses demand forecasts to dramatically reduce its inventory costs (Doan 1999). Nonstop Solutions uses Longs sales data to forecast sales patterns for each of its 362 retail stores. The Nonstop algorithm, based on research by its founder, Professor Hau Lee of Stanford University, factors in variables such as the season and demand trends for individual stores. It then translates these demand forecasts into inventory recommendations for each store for individual pharmaceuticals, dosages, and bottle sizes. Armed with this information, Longs Drug Stores was able to sharply reduce inventories at its central warehouse and its stores. For example, it was able to reduce its inventory of Xanax, an antianxiety drug, from 26 days' worth of orders to 6.7 days' worth. This single change reduced the amount of cash devoted to inventory by $15,210.

In addition to increasing profits, the Nonstop system allows pharmacists to concentrate more on customer service and less on inventory management. For example, one pharmacist who was no longer tied up in checking his inventory began developing a program for in-store cholesterol screenings.

---

price, it will be rationed by other means, such as waiting times, that are often inconvenient for consumers. In addition, careful analyses of consumer use of services have convinced most analysts that medical goods and services should not be free. If care was truly costless for consumers, they would use it until it offered them no additional value. Today this understanding is reflected in the public and private insurance plans of most nations.

Care cannot really be free. Someone must pay, somehow. Modern healthcare requires the services of highly skilled professionals, complex and elaborate equipment, and specialized supplies. Even the resources for which there is no charge represent a cost to someone.

6.1.1 Indirect Payments and Insurance

Because the burden of healthcare costs falls primarily on an unfortunate few, health insurance is common. Insurance creates another use for demand analyses. To design sensible insurance plans we need to understand the public's valuation of services. Insurance plans seek to identify benefits the public is willing to pay for. The public may pay directly (called an out-of-pocket payment) or indirectly. Indirect payments can take the form of health insurance premiums, taxes, wage reductions, or higher prices for other products. Understanding the public's valuation is especially important in the healthcare sector because indirect payments are so common. When consumers pay directly, valuation is not very important (except for making revenue forecasts). Right or wrong, a consumer who refuses to buy a $7.50 bottle of aspirin from an airport vendor because it is "too expensive" is making a clear statement about value. In contrast, a Medicare patient who thinks coronary artery bypass graft surgery is a good buy at a cost of $1,000 is not providing us with useful information. The surgery costs more than $30,000, but the patient and taxpayers pay most of the bill indirectly. Because so much medical care is purchased indirectly, with the assistance of public or private insurance, it is often difficult to assess whether the values of goods and services are as large as their costs.

6.2 Why Demand for Healthcare Is Complex

The demand for medical care is more complex than the demand for many other goods for four reasons.

1. The price of care often depends on insurance coverage. Insurance has powerful effects on demand and makes analysis more complex.
2. Healthcare decisions are typically quite perplexing. Consumers would prefer to be healthy and use no medical services. Medical services have value largely because of their impact on health. The links between medical care and health outcomes are often difficult to ascertain at the population level (where the average impact of care is what matters) and stunningly complex at the individual level (where what happens to me is what matters). Forced to make hard choices, consumers may make bad choices.
3. This complexity contributes to consumers' poor information about costs and benefits of care. Such "rational ignorance" is natural. Most consumers will not have to make most healthcare choices, and it makes no sense to be prepared to do so.
4. The net effect of complexity and consumer ignorance is that producers have significant influence on demand. Quite naturally, consumers turn to healthcare professionals for advice. Unfortunately, because they are human, professionals' choices are likely to reflect their values and incentives as well as those of their patients.

Demand is complicated by itself. To keep things simple, we will first examine the demand for medical goods and services where insurance and the guidance of healthcare professionals play no role. The demand for over-the-counter pharmaceuticals, such as aspirin, is an example of this "simple" case. We will then add insurance to the mix but keep professional advice out. The demand for dental prophylaxis will be our example in this case. Finally, we will add the role of professional advice.

6.3 Demand Without Insurance and Healthcare Professionals

In principle, a consumer's decision to buy a particular good or service reflects a maddening array of considerations. For example, a consumer with a headache who is considering buying a bottle of aspirin must compare his perceptions of its benefit to his other choices. Those other choices might include taking a nap, going for a walk, taking another nonprescription analgesic, and consulting a physician.

Economic models of demand radically simplify descriptions of consumer choices by stressing three key relationships:

1. The impact of changes in the price of a good or service
2. Changes in the prices of related goods or services
3. Changes in consumer incomes on the amount purchased

This simplification is valuable to firms and policymakers, who cannot change much besides prices and incomes. This focus can be misleading, however, if it obscures the potential impact of public information campaigns (including advertising).

6.3.1 Changes in Price

The fundamental prediction of demand theory is that the quantity demanded will decrease when the price of a good or service rises. The quantity demanded may decrease because some consumers buy smaller amounts of a product (as might be the case with analgesics) or because a smaller proportion of the population chooses to buy a product (as might be the case with dental prophylaxis). Figure 6.1 illustrates this sort of relationship. On demand curve D_1 a price reduction from P_1 to P_2 increases the quantity demanded from Q_1 to Q_2.

Figure 6.1 also illustrates a shift in demand. At each price, demand curve D_2 indicates a lower quantity demanded than demand curve D_1. (Alternatively, at each volume, willingness to pay will be smaller with D_2.) This sort of shift might be due to a drop in income, a drop in the price of a substitute, an increase in the price of a complement, a change in demographics or consumer information, or other factors.

Demand curves can also be interpreted to mean prices will have to be cut to increase the sales volume. Consumers who are not willing to pay what the product now costs may enter the market at a lower price, or current consumers may use more of the product at a lower price.

Like Figure 6.1, Figure 6.2 illustrates a shift in demand. In Figure 6.2, however, the demand curves are not straight lines.

FIGURE 6.1

Linear Demand

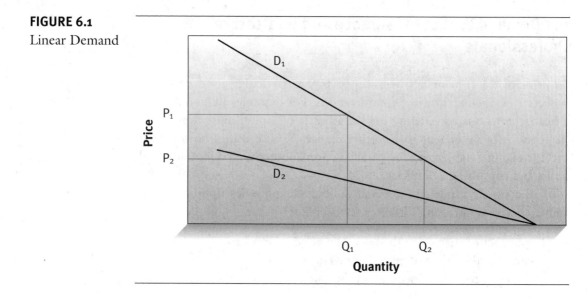

Demand curves are important economic tools. Analysts use statistical techniques to estimate how much the quantity demanded will change if the price of the product, income, or other factors change.

Substitution explains why demand curves generally slope down, that is, why consumption of a product usually falls if its price rises. Substitutes exist for most goods and services. When the price of a product is higher than that of its substitute, more people choose the substitute. Substitutes for aspirin include taking a nap, going for a walk, taking another nonprescription analgesic, and consulting a physician. If there are close substitutes, changes in a product's price could lead to large changes in consumption. If none of the alternatives are close substitutes, changes in a product's price will lead to smaller changes in consumption. Taking another nonprescription analgesic is a close substitute for taking aspirin, so we would anticipate that consumers would be sensitive to changes in the price of aspirin.

Substitution is not the only result of a change in price, of course. When the price of a good or service falls, the consumer has more money to spend on all goods and services. Most of the time this "income effect" reinforces the "substitution effect," so we can predict with confidence that a price reduction will cause consumers to buy more of that good. In a few cases, things get murkier. A rise in the wage rate, for example, increases the income you would forgo by reducing your work week. At first blush, you might expect a higher wage rate would reduce your demand for time off. At the same time, though, a higher wage rate increases your income, which may mean more money for travel and leisure activities, increasing the amount of time you want off. In these cases empirical work is necessary to predict the impact of a change in prices.

Two points about price sensitivity need to be made here. First, a general perception that use of most goods and services will fall if prices rise

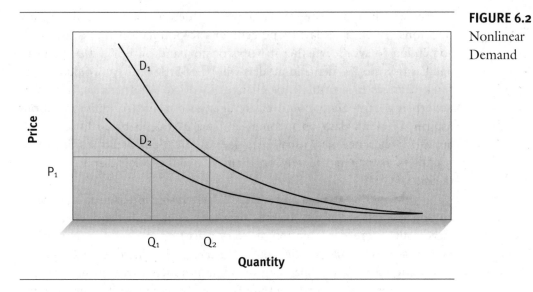

FIGURE 6.2
Nonlinear
Demand

is a useful notion to keep tucked away. Second, managers need more precise guidance. How much will sales increase if I reduce prices by 10 percent? Will my total revenue rise or fall as a result? To answer these questions takes empirical analysis. Fleshing out general notions about price sensitivity with estimates is one of the tasks of economic analysis. We also need an agreed-upon terminology to talk about how much the quantity demanded will change in response to a change in income, the price of the product, or the prices of other products. Economists describe these relationships in terms of elasticities, which we will talk more about later.

6.3.2 Factors Other Than Price

Changes in factors other than the price of a product shift the entire demand curve. Changes in beliefs about the productivity of a good or service, preferences, the prices of related goods and services, and income can shift the demand curve.

Consumers' beliefs about the health effects of products are obviously central to discussions of demand. Few people want aspirin for its own sake. The demand for aspirin, as for most medical goods and services, depends on consumers' expectations about its effects on their health. These expectations have two dimensions. One dimension depends on consumers' beliefs about their own health. If they believe they are healthy, they are unlikely to purchase goods and services to improve their health. The other dimension depends on their perception of how much a product will improve health. If I have a headache but do not believe that aspirin will relieve it, I will not be willing to buy it. Health status and beliefs about the capacity of goods and services to improve health underpin demand.

Demand is a useful construct only if consumer preferences are stable enough to allow us to predict responses to price and income changes and if price and income changes are important determinants of consumption decisions. If on Tuesday 14 percent of the population thinks aspirin is something to avoid (whether it works or not) and on Friday that percentage has risen to 24, demand models will be of little use. We would need to track changes in attitude, not changes in price. Alternatively, if routine advertising campaigns could easily change consumers' opinions about aspirin, tracking data on incomes and prices would be of little use. It appears preferences are usually stable enough for demand studies to be useful, so managers can rely on them in making pricing and marketing decisions.

Changes in income and wealth usually result in changes in demand. In principle, an increase in income or wealth could shift the demand curve either out (more consumption at every price) or in (less consumption at every price). Overall spending on healthcare clearly increases with income (Di Matteo 2003), but spending on some products falls with income. For example, emergency department use falls for consumers with higher incomes (Bernstein 2008). For the most part, however, consumers with larger budgets buy more healthcare products.

Changes in the prices of related goods also shift demand curves. Related goods are substitutes (products used instead of the product in question) and complements (products used in conjunction with the product in question). A substitute need not be a perfect substitute; in some cases it is simply an alternative. For example, ibuprofen is a substitute for aspirin. A reduction in the price of a substitute usually shifts the demand curve in (reduced willingness to pay at every volume). If the price of ibuprofen fell, some consumers would be tempted to switch from aspirin to ibuprofen and the demand for aspirin would shift in. Conversely, an increase in the price of a substitute usually shifts the demand curve out (increased willingness to pay at every volume). If the price of ibuprofen rose, some consumers would be tempted to switch from ibuprofen to aspirin and the demand for aspirin would shift out.

6.4 Demand with Insurance

Insurance changes demand by reducing the price of covered goods and services. For example, a consumer whose dental insurance plan covers 80 percent of the cost of a routine examination will need to pay only $10 instead of the full $50. The volume of routine examinations will usually increase as a result of an increase in insurance coverage, primarily because a higher proportion of the covered population will seek this form of preventive care. The response will not typically be large, however. Most consumers will not change their decisions to seek care because prices have changed. But managers should

Case 6.1   MinuteClinics

"MinuteClinic healthcare centers are an answer to consumers' overwhelming demand for more patient-centric healthcare," said Michael Howe, CEO of MinuteClinic. "As more patients look to take control of their healthcare options, we provide a fast, convenient, and affordable service for common maladies that is available seven days a week."

MinuteClinic started in 2000 and now has more than 500 locations. Its clinics are staffed by nurse practitioners and physician assistants, rather than physicians. The clinics are open seven days a week, and appointments are not needed. The nurse practitioners and physician assistants diagnose, treat, and write prescriptions for a variety of common illnesses. Most clinics are in CVS pharmacies.

MinuteClinic started in Minnesota. One wintry weekend in 1999, Rick Krieger took his son to an urgent care center in Minneapolis to get a strep throat test. After a two-hour wait, his son finally got his test. Krieger thought there had to be a quicker, more convenient way of getting basic medical care. A year later Krieger and his partners started their first retail clinic.

Of course, not everyone thinks MinuteClinics are a good idea. In a written statement, Boston Mayor Thomas Menino launched a public campaign in opposition to a plan to open multiple MinuteClinics in Boston. He said, "Limited-service medical clinics run by merchants in for-profit corporations will seriously compromise quality of care and hygiene. Allowing retailers to make money off of sick people is wrong." Normand Deschene, president and CEO of Lowell General Hospital, voiced concerns that the clinics could jeopardize the continuity of care. "I have concerns about patients being taken care of by someone without knowledge of their history." At Lowell General patients with minor problems are seen in the urgent care section of the emergency room. "The clinics are the latest big example of how you could think about consumers and what their needs are, rather than a healthcare system exclusively designed around the needs of providers," said Margaret Laws of the California Health Care Foundation (Freudenheim 2008).

Discussion questions:
- For what products is a MinuteClinic a substitute?
- For what products is it a complement?
- In what sense is a MinuteClinic designed to meet the needs of patients?
- Do you share Mayor Menino's concerns?
- Why might he be right?
- Why might he be wrong?

FIGURE 6.3

The Impact of
Insurance on
Demand

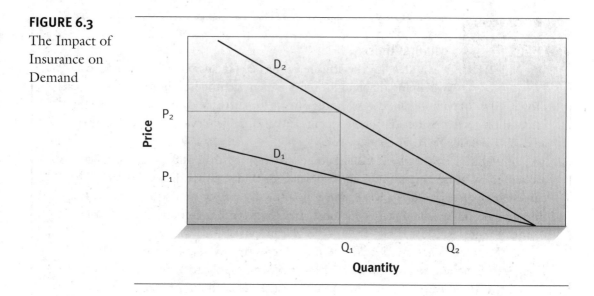

recognize that some consumers will respond to price changes caused by insurance. (We will develop tools for describing responses to price changes and review the evidence on this score in the next chapter.)

Figure 6.3 depicts standard responses to increases in insurance. An increase in insurance (a higher share of the population covered or a higher share of the bill covered) rotates the demand curve from D_1 to D_2. As a result, the quantity demanded will rise from Q_1 to Q_2 if the price remains at P_1. Or, if the quantity remains at Q_1, the price could rise from P_1 to P_2.

For provider organizations, an increase in insurance represents an opportunity to increase prices and margins. The rotation of D_2 has made it steeper, meaning that demand has become less sensitive to price. As demand becomes less sensitive to price, profit-maximizing firms will seek higher margins. (Higher margins mean the cost of production will represent a smaller share of what consumers pay for a product.) Higher prices and increased quantity mean expansion of unmanaged insurance will result in substantial increases in spending.

6.5 Demand with Advice from Providers

Consumers are often rationally ignorant about the healthcare system and the particular decisions they need to make. They are ignorant because medical decisions are complex, because they are unfamiliar with their options, because they lack the skills and information they need to compare their options, and because they lack time to make a considered judgment. This ignorance is rational because consumers do not know what choices they will have to make, because the cost of acquiring skills and information is high,

Sidebar 6.2 Increased Cost Sharing

Demand theory implies that having patients pay a larger share of the bill (usually termed *increased cost sharing*) should reduce consumption of care. Does it? A landmark study by the RAND Corporation tells us that it does (Manning et al. 1987). The RAND Health Insurance Experiment randomly assigned consumers to 15 different health plans in six locations and then tracked their use of care (see Table 6.1). Its fee-for-service sites had coinsurance rates of 0 percent, 25 percent, 50 percent, and 95 percent. The health plans fully covered expenses above *stop loss limits* (the maximum amount a consumer would have to pay out of pocket), which varied from 5 percent to 15 percent of income. Spending was substantially lower for consumers who shared in the cost of their care. Increasing the coinsurance rate (the share of the bill that consumers pay) from 0 percent to 25 percent reduced total spending by nearly a fifth. This reduction had minimal effects on health.

TABLE 6.1
Effect of Coinsurance Rate

Coinsurance Rate	Spending	Any Use of Care	Hospital Admission
0%	$750	87%	10%
25%	$617	79%	8%
50%	$573	77%	7%
95%	$540	68%	8%

Costs were lower because consumers had fewer contacts with the healthcare system. The experiment went on for a number of years, and the suspicion that reducing use of care would increase spending later was not borne out. Based on the results of this study, virtually all insurance plans now incorporate some form of cost sharing for care initiated by patients.

and because the benefits of acquiring these skills and information are unknown.

Consumers routinely deal with situations in which they are ignorant. Few consumers really know whether their car needs a new constant velocity joint, whether the roof should be replaced or repaired, or whether they should sell their stock in Cerner Corporation. Of course, consumers know they are ignorant. They often seek an *agent*, someone who is knowledgeable and can offer advice that advances the consumers' interests. Most people with medical problems choose a physician to be their agent.

Using an agent reduces, but does not eliminate, the problems associated with ignorance. Agents sometimes take advantage of principals (the ignorant consumers they represent). Taking advantage can range from out-and-out fraud (e.g., lying to sell a worthless insurance policy) to simple shirking (e.g., failing to check the accuracy of ads for a property). If consumers can identify poor agent performance, fairly simple remedies further reduce the problems associated with ignorance. In many cases an agent's reputation is of paramount importance, so agents have a strong incentive to please principals. In other cases simply delaying payment until a project has been successfully completed substantially reduces agency problems.

The most difficult problems arise when consumers have difficulty distinguishing bad outcomes from bad performance on the part of an agent. This is a fairly common problem. Did your house take a long time to sell because the market weakened unexpectedly or because your agent recommended that you set the price too high? Was your baby born via cesarean section to preserve her health or to preserve your physician's weekend plans? Most contracts with agents are designed to minimize these problems by aligning the interests of the principal and the agent. For example, real estate agents earn a share of a property's sale price, so that both the agent and the seller profit when the property is sold quickly at a high price. In similar fashion, earnings of mutual fund managers are commonly based on the total assets they manage, so managers and investors profit when the value of the mutual fund increases.

Agency models have several implications for our understanding of demand. First, what consumers demand may depend on incentives for providers. Agency models suggest that changes in the amount paid to providers, the way providers are paid, or providers' profits may change their recommendations for consumers. For example, consumers may respond to a lower price for generic drugs only because pharmacists have financial incentives to recommend them. Second, provider incentives will affect consumption of some goods and services more than others. Provider recommendations will not affect patients' initial decisions to seek care. And where standards of care are clear and generally accepted, providers are less apt to change their recommendations when their incentives change. When there is a consensus about standards of care, providers who change their recommendations in response to financial incentives risk denial of payment, identification as a low-quality provider, or even malpractice suits. Third, patients with chronic illnesses are often quite knowledgeable about the therapies they prefer. When patients have firm preferences, agency is likely to have less effect on demand. In short, agency makes the demand for medical care more complex.

Most important, agency is one of the factors that makes managed care necessary. (That insurance plans must protect consumers from virtually all of the costs of some very expensive procedures, so out-of-pocket costs need to fall to near zero, is the other main factor.) If all the parties to a healthcare transaction had all the same information, expenditures could be limited simply by changing consumer out-of-pocket payments. In many cases, though, provider incentives need to be aligned with consumer goals. (Of course, health plans also have an agency relationship with beneficiaries, and nothing guarantees plans will be perfect agents.) Most of the features of managed care address the agency problem in one way or another. Global payments for services and capitation are designed to give physicians incentives to recommend no more care than is really necessary. Primary care gatekeepers are supposed to monitor recommendations for specialty services (from which they derive no financial benefit).

6.6 Conclusion

Demand is one of the central ideas of economics, and managers need to understand the basics of demand. In most cases, consumption of a product falls when its price is increased, and studies of healthcare products confirm this generalization. An understanding of this relationship between price and quantity is part of effective management. Without it managers cannot predict sales, revenues, or profits.

To make accurate forecasts, managers also must be aware of the effects of factors they do not control. Demand for their products will be higher when the price of complements is lower or the price of substitutes is higher. In most cases, demand will be higher in areas with higher incomes. We will explore how to make forecasts in more detail in Chapter 7.

The demand for healthcare products is complex. Insurance and professional advice have significant effects on demand. Insurance means there are three prices: the out-of-pocket price the consumer pays, the price the insurer pays, and the price the provider charges. The quantity demanded will usually fall when out-of-pocket prices rise, but may not change when the other prices do. Because professional advice is important in consumers' healthcare decisions, the incentives professionals face can influence consumption of some products. How and how much professionals are paid can affect their recommendations, and recognition of this has helped spur the shift to managed care. To change patterns of consumption, managers may need to change incentives for patients and providers.

Homework

6.1 Is the idea of demand useful in healthcare, given the important role of agents?

6.2 Should medical services be free? Justify your answer.

6.3 Why might a consumer be "rationally ignorant" about the proper therapy for gall stones?

6.4 Why do demand curves slope down (i.e., sales volume usually rises at lower prices)?

6.5 Why would consumers ever choose insurance plans with large deductibles?

6.6 During the last five years average daily occupancy at Autumn Acres nursing home has slid from 125 to 95 even though Autumn Acres has cut its daily rate from $125 to $115. Do these data suggest that occupancy would have been higher if Autumn Acres had raised its rates? What changes in nonprice demand factors might explain this? (There have been no changes in supply. The number of nursing home beds in the area has not changed during this period.)

6.7 Your hospital is considering opening a satellite urgent care center about five miles from your main campus. You have been charged with gathering demographic information that might affect the demand for the center's services. What data are likely to be relevant?

6.8 How would each of the following changes affect the demand curve for acupuncture?

a. The price of an acupuncture session increases.

b. There is a reduction in back problems due to sessions on stretching on the *Oprah Winfrey Show*.

c. Medicare reduces the copayment for acupuncture from $20 to $10.

d. The surgeon general issues a warning that back surgery is ineffective.

e. Medicare stops covering back surgery.

6.9 Your boss has asked you to describe how the demand for an over-the-counter sinus medication would change in the following situations. Assuming the price does not change, forecast whether the sales volume will go up, remain constant, or go down.

a. The local population increases.

b. A wet spring leads to a bumper crop of ragweed.

c. Factory closings lead to a drop in the area's average income.

d. A competing product with a different formula is found to be unsafe.

e. A research study is published showing that the medication causes severe dizziness.

f. The price of another sinus medication drops.

6.10 A community has four residents. The table below shows the number of dental visits each will have. Calculate the total quantity that will be demanded at each price, then graph the relationship between price and total quantity, with total quantity on the horizontal axis.

Price	Abe's Quantity	Beth's Quantity	Cal's Quantity	Don's Quantity
$40	0	0	0	1
$30	0	1	0	1
$20	0	1	0	2
$10	1	2	1	2
$0	1	2	1	3

6.11 A clinic focuses on three services: counseling for teens and young adults, smoking cessation, and counseling for young parents. An analyst has developed a forecast of the number of visits each group will make at different prices. Calculate the total quantity that will be demanded at each price, then graph the relationship between price and total quantity, putting total quantity on the horizontal axis.

Price	Teen Counseling	Smoking Cessation	Parent Counseling
$80	10	0	0
$60	15	1	0
$40	20	2	0
$20	40	4	6
$0	50	6	8

6.12 The price-quantity relationship has been estimated for the new prostate cancer blood test: $Q = 4,000 - 20 \times P$. Use a spreadsheet to calculate the quantity demanded and total spending for prices ranging from $200 to $0, using $50 increments. For each $50 drop in price calculate the change in revenue, the change in volume, and the additional revenue per unit. Call the additional revenue per unit marginal revenue.

6.13 A physical therapy clinic faces a demand equation of $Q = 200 - 1.5 \times P$, where Q is sessions per month and P is the price per session.
   a. The clinic currently charges $80. What is its sales volume and revenue at this price?
   b. If the clinic raised its price to $90, what would happen to volume and revenue?
   c. If the clinic lowered its price to $70, what would happen to volume and revenue?

6.14 Researchers have concluded that the demand for annual preventive clinic visits by children with asthma equals $1 + 0.00004 \times Y - 0.04 \times P$. In this equation Y represents family income and P represents price.
   a. Calculate how many visits a child with a family income of $100,000 will make at prices of $200, $150, $100, $50, and $0. If you predict that visits will be less than zero, convert your answer to a zero.
   b. Now repeat your calculations for a child with a family income of $35,000.
   c. How do your predictions for the two children differ?
   d. Assume that the market price of a preventive visit is $100. Does this seem like a fair system to you? What fairness criteria are you using?
   e. Would your answer change if the surgeon general recommended that every child with asthma have at least one preventive visit each year?

Chapter Glossary

Complement. A product used in conjunction with another product

Copayment. A fee that the patient must pay in addition to the amount paid by insurance

Cost sharing. The general term for direct payments to providers by insurance beneficiaries. Deductibles, copayments, and coinsurance are forms of cost sharing

Demand. The amounts of a good or service that will be purchased at different prices when all other factors are held constant

Demand curve. A tool for describing how much consumers are willing to buy at different prices

Demand shift. A shift that occurs when a factor other than price (e.g., consumer incomes) changes

Increase or decrease in demand. A shift in the entire list of amounts that will be purchased at different prices

Market demand. The sum of the demands of all consumers in a market

Market system. A system that uses prices to ration goods and services

Moral hazard. The incentive to use additional care that having insurance creates

Out-of-pocket price. The amount of money a consumer herself pays for a good or service

Quantity demanded. The amount of a good or service that will be purchased at a specific price when all other factors are held constant

Shift in demand. A shift that occurs when a factor other than price of the product itself (e.g., consumer incomes) changes

Substitute. A product used instead of another product

References

Bernstein, D. P. 2008. "Factors Impacting Emergency Department Use." [Online information; retrieved 12/17/08.] http://papers.ssrn.com/sol3/papers.cfm?abstract_id=1284582.

Di Matteo, L. 2003. "The Income Elasticity of Health Care Spending: A Comparison of Parametric and Nonparametric Approaches." *The European Journal of Health Economics* 4 (1): 20–29.

Doan, A. 1999. "Vitamin Efficiency." *Forbes* 64 (11): 176–86.

Freudenheim, M. 2008. "Wal-Mart Will Expand In-Store Medical Clinics." [Online article; retrieved 4/20/08.] www.nytimes.com/2008/02/07/business/07clinic.html.

Manning, W. G., A. Leibowitz, M. S. Marquis, J. P. Newhouse, N. Duan, and E. B. Keeler. 1987. "Health Insurance and the Demand for Medical Care: Evidence from a Randomized Experiment." *American Economic Review* 77 (3): 251–77.

ELASTICITIES

Learning Objectives

After reading this chapter, students will be able to:

- **calculate** an arc elasticity,
- **use** elasticities to describe economic data,
- **apply** elasticities to make simple forecasts, and
- **use** elasticity terms appropriately.

Key Concepts

- Economists use elasticities to avoid confusion about units.
- An elasticity is the percentage change in one variable that is associated with a 1 percent change in another.
- Elasticities allow quick calculations of the effects of strategic choices.
- Managers can use elasticities to forecast sales.
- To avoid ambiguities, use arc elasticities (which use the average of the starting and ending values as the denominator of percentage change calculations).
- An income elasticity of demand is the percentage change in the quantity demanded that is associated with a 1 percent change in consumer income.
- A price elasticity of demand is the percentage change in the quantity demanded that is associated with a 1 percent change in the price of a product.
- A cross-price elasticity is the percentage change in the quantity demanded that is associated with a 1 percent change in the price of a substitute or complement.

7.1 Introduction

Elasticities are valuable tools for managers. Armed only with basic marketing data and reasonable estimates about elasticities, managers can make sales, revenue, and marginal revenue forecasts. In addition, elasticities are ideal for analyzing "what if" questions. What will happen to revenues if we raise prices by

2 percent? What will happen to our sales if the price of a substitute drops by 3 percent?

Elasticities reduce confusion in descriptions. For example, suppose the price of a 500-tablet bottle of generic ibuprofen rose from $7.50 to $8.00. Someone who was seeking to downplay the size of this increase (or someone whose focus was on the cost per tablet) would say that the price rose from 1.5 cents to 1.6 cents per tablet. Describing this change in percentage terms would eliminate any confusion about price per bottle or price per tablet, but there is still a potential source of confusion. The change could be described as an increase of 6.67 percent (by dividing the increase, 50 cents, into $7.50) or 6.25 percent (by dividing the increase into $8.00).

To avoid confusion in calculating percentages, economists recommend two courses of action. One is to be very explicit about the values used to calculate percentage changes. For example, one might say that the price increase to $8.00 represents a 6.67 percent increase from the starting value of $7.50. In our view, the best course of action is to use the average of the starting and ending values to calculate percentage changes, because that avoids some complications that may confuse the unwary. In this case, using the average price of $7.75 to calculate the percentages means that only one answer is possible: Prices increased 6.45 percent.

7.2 Elasticities

An *elasticity* is the percentage change in one variable associated with a 1 percent change in another. For example, Newhouse and Phelps (1976) used statistical techniques to estimate that the income elasticity for physician visits was 0.04. The base for this estimate is average income, so an income 1 percent above the average is associated with an average level of physician visits that is 0.04 percent above average. As we shall see, these apparently esoteric estimates can be quite valuable to managers.

First we need to learn a little more about elasticities. Economists routinely calculate three demand elasticities:

1. **income elasticity**: the percentage change in the quantity demanded that is associated with a 1 percent change in consumer income
2. **price elasticity**: the percentage change in the quantity demanded that is associated with a 1 percent change in a product's price
3. **cross-price elasticity**: the percentage change in the quantity demanded that is associated with a 1 percent change in the price of a substitute or complement

All these elasticities can be represented as ratios of percentage changes. For example, the income elasticity of demand for visits would equal the ratio of the percentage change in visits (dQ/Q) associated with a given percentage change in income (dY/Y). (The mathematical terms dQ and dY identify small changes in consumption and income.) So, the formula for an income elasticity would be $E_Y = (dQ/Q)/(dY/Y)$. The formula for a price elasticity would be $E_P = (dQ/Q)/(dP/P)$, and the formula for cross-price elasticity would be $E_R = (dQ/Q)/(dR/R)$. (A cross-price elasticity measures the response of demand to changes in the price of a substitute or complement, so R is the price of a related product.)

Now recall that the Newhouse and Phelps estimate of the income elasticity for physician visits is 0.04. This implies that $0.04 = (dQ/Q)/(dY/Y)$. Suppose we wanted to know how much higher than average visits per person would be in an area where the average income is 2 percent higher than the national average. As we are considering a case in which dY/Y = 0.02, we multiply both sides of the equation by 0.02 and find that visits should be 0.0008 (0.08 percent) higher in an area with income 2 percent above the national average. From the perspective of a working manager, what matters is the conclusion that visits will only be slightly higher in the wealthier area.

7.3 Income Elasticities

Consumption of most healthcare products increases with income, but only slightly. As Table 7.1 shows, consumption of healthcare products appears to increase more slowly than income. As a result, healthcare spending will represent a smaller proportion of income among high-income consumers than among low-income consumers.

7.4 Price Elasticities of Demand

The price elasticity of demand is even more useful, because prices depend on choices managers make. Estimates of the price elasticity of demand will guide pricing and contracting decisions, as Chapter 9 explores in more detail. Managers need to be careful in using the price elasticity of demand for three

TABLE 7.1
Selected Estimates of the Income Elasticity of Demand

Source	Date	Variable	Point Estimate
Rosett and Huang	1973	Spending per person	0.25 to 0.45
Newhouse and Phelps	1976	Hospital admissions	0.02 to 0.04
		Physician visits	0.01 to 0.04

reasons. First, because the price elasticity of demand is almost always negative, we need a special vocabulary to describe the responsiveness of demand to price. For example, –3.00 is a smaller number than –1.00, but –3.00 implies that demand is more responsive to changes in prices (a 1 percent rise in prices results in a 3 percent drop in sales rather than a 1 percent drop in sales). Second, changes in prices affect revenues directly and indirectly, via changes in quantity. Managers need to keep this in mind when using the price elasticity of demand. Third, there are two very different price elasticities of demand managers need to think about: the overall price elasticity of demand and the price elasticity of demand for his or her firm's products.

Economists usually speak of price elasticities of demand (but not other elasticities) as being *inelastic* or *elastic*. When a 1 percent increase in price results in a less than 1 percent reduction in the quantity demanded, the price elasticity of demand will be between 0.00 and –1.00, and demand is said to be *inelastic*. When a 1 percent increase in price results in a more than 1 percent reduction in the quantity demanded, the price elasticity of demand will be smaller than –1.00, and demand is said to be *elastic*.

It is important to recognize that inelastic demand does not mean consumption will be unaffected by price changes. Suppose that, in forecasting the demand response to a 3 percent price cut, we use an elasticity of –0.20. Predicting that sales will drop by 0.6 percent, this elasticity implies that demand is inelastic but not unresponsive. Recall that a price elasticity of demand equals the ratio of the percentage change in quantity that is associated with a percentage change in price, or $(dQ/Q)/(dP/P)$. Using this formula and our elasticity estimate gives us $-0.20 = (dQ/Q)/-0.03$. After solving for the percentage change in quantity, we forecast that a 3 percent price cut will increase consumption by 0.006 (or 0.6 percent), which is equal to -0.20×-0.03. Table 7.2 shows that the demand for medical care is usually inelastic.

7.5 Using Elasticities

Elasticities are useful forecasting tools. With an estimate of the price elasticity of demand, a manager can quickly estimate the impact of a price cut on

TABLE 7.2

Selected Estimates of the Price Elasticity of Demand

Source	Date	Variable	Point Estimate
Manning et al.	1987	Total spending	–0.17 to –0.22
Newhouse and Phelps	1976	Hospital admissions	–0.02 to –0.04
		Physician visits	–0.08

Case 7.1 Mental Health Parity

Colleen McGuire was passionate in her presentation to the board.

"Our insurance plan should provide the same coverage for mental health services as other medical services. It's the right thing to do and it's good business. If your employees or dependents have untreated mental health problems, your employees become less productive and waste money getting treated for other stuff."

"Thank you, Colleen," said Kerry Landrum, our CEO. "This is an important question for us, and you can be sure the Benefits Committee will carefully consider it." After Colleen left the room Kerry turned to Jordan Hewitt, our director of human resources, and said, "Jordan, what's your take on this?"

"There are actually two questions here," said Jordan. "First, how elastic is the demand for ambulatory mental health services? How much will use of mental health services increase if coverage improves? Second, how effective is mental health care? This turns out to be the more important question, because good mental health care can have such powerful effects.

"Now, a number of studies have concluded that use of mental health services is more price sensitive than use of other ambulatory care. Analyses of ambulatory mental health services have found elasticities ranging from −0.44 to −1.00. These results could be statistical flukes. Consumers who expect to use mental health services may choose insurance plans that offer generous coverage for mental health services. However, RAND Corporation researchers used data from the Health Insurance Experiment, which randomly assigned respondents to insurance plans, to resolve this issue (Keeler, Manning, and Wells 1988).

"The RAND analysis generally confirmed that the demand for mental health services is more price sensitive than demand for general ambulatory medical services. Demand for each is inelastic, but the elasticity for mental health services is −0.8 and the elasticity for other outpatient services is −0.3. Most consumers will not use any mental health services, but plans that offer generous mental health benefits will cost more. We can't ignore this."

"I'm confused," said Addison Wells, an internist on our board. "In 2006 Goldman and his colleagues published a study showing that Bill Clinton's 1999 executive order requiring mental health parity for federal workers had little effect on spending. How could that be? Real life appears to be contradicting the RAND study."

"I'm sure the plans for federal employees used managed care techniques to control spending," Jordan Hewitt jumped in. "And mental health spending isn't the issue. The issues are what happens to other healthcare spending and what happens to our workers. I'm pretty sure there's good evidence showing that effective mental health treatment can reduce other costs and improve productivity."

(continued)

Case 7.1 continued

Discussion questions:
- Why does it matter whether demand for mental health services is more elastic than demand for other services?
- The price elasticity of demand for ambulatory mental health services appears to be about –0.8, and the price elasticity for general ambulatory medical services appears to be about –0.3. How much would spending increase for each type of care if copays were cut from $40 to $25?
- What managed care techniques do insurers use to control spending?
- Is there evidence that better treatment of mental health problems reduces other spending?
- Is there evidence that it improves productivity?
- What is your recommendation to the Benefits Committee?

sales and revenues. As we noted earlier though, managers need to use the correct elasticity. Most estimates of the overall price elasticity of demand fall between –0.10 and –0.40. For the market as a whole, the demand for healthcare products is typically inelastic. For individual firms, in contrast, demand is usually elastic. The reason is quite simple. Most healthcare products have few close substitutes, but the products of one healthcare organization represent close substitutes for the products of another.

The price elasticity of demand individual firms face typically depends on the overall price elasticity and the firm's market share. So, if the price elasticity of demand for hospital admissions is –0.17 and a hospital has a 12 percent share of the market, the hospital needs to anticipate that it faces a price elasticity of –0.17/0.12, or –1.42. This rule of thumb need not hold exactly, but there is good evidence that individual firms confront elastic demand. For example, Lee and Hadley (1981) estimated that the price elasticity of demand for the services of individual physicians ranged from –2.80 to –5.07. Indeed, as we will show in Chapter 8, profit-maximizing firms should set prices high enough that demand for their products is elastic.

Armed with a reasonable estimate of the price elasticity of demand, we will now predict the impact of a 5 percent price cut on volume. If the price elasticity faced by a physician firm were –2.80, a 5 percent price cut should increase the number of visits by 14 percent, which is the product of –0.05 and –2.80. (A prudent manager will recognize that her best guess about the price elasticity will not be exactly right and repeat the calculations with other values. For example, if the price elasticity is really –1.40, volume will increase

Case 7.2	**Reducing Waiting Time**

One of the few determinants of demand that healthcare managers can control is waiting time. There is ample evidence that long waits discourage patients and drive up costs. Acton (1975) estimated that the elasticity of demand with respect to waiting time was −0.96 in clinics (where waits tended to be long) and −0.25 in physicians' offices (where waits tended to be shorter). This suggests that reducing waits by 10 percent could increase volume by 3 to 10 percent. In an environment in which many providers would like to add patients, reducing waits represents a strategy worth considering.

The Women's Medicine Center of Charleston Area Medical Center used a Six Sigma approach to improve patient access. As a result the wait for a new appointment dropped from 38 days to 8 days, and the average time patients spent in the clinic dropped from 3.2 hours to 1.5 hours. Not surprisingly, business improved dramatically. Volumes and revenue increased by over 50 percent, and patient satisfaction increased sharply (Bush et al. 2007).

Six Sigma is a structured performance improvement approach that stresses defining the organization's problem from the perspective of internal and external customers, measuring key aspects of performance, analyzing the data, and putting in place a plan for improvement. The Women's Medicine Center added clinic sessions, changed the scheduling process, simplified how patients moved through the clinic, and added a part-time nurse practitioner and a part-time nurse midwife to the staff.

More volume may not be the only benefit of reducing waiting time. Long waits for patients often mean long waits for staff as well. Another hospital reported that new procedures in its emergency department reduced waits by two-thirds. Not only did satisfaction scores nearly double but also cost per visit fell by 12 percent, saving more than $422,000 (Anonymous 1997). At the risk of belaboring the obvious, changes that increase satisfaction while reducing costs will generally improve a manager's career prospects.

Discussion questions:
* Acton's estimates suggest that demand is more sensitive to waiting time than to out-of-pocket price. Why might that be the case?
* How much of a percentage change is a reduction from 3.2 hours to 1.5 hours?
* Just for the sake of argument, assume that the entire increase in volume is due to the reduction in visit lengths. What elasticity of demand with respect to visit length do the data for the Women's Medicine Center imply?
* Why would waits for patients result in waits for staff?

by 7 percent. Or, if the price elasticity is really –4.20, volume will increase by 21 percent.)

How much will revenues change if we cut prices by 5 percent and the price elasticity is –2.80? Obviously revenues will rise by less than volume because we have reduced prices. A rough, easily calculated estimate of the change in revenues is the percentage change in prices plus the percentage change in volume. Prices will fall by 5 percent and quantity will rise by 7 to 21 percent, so revenues should rise by approximately 2 to 16 percent. Our baseline estimate is that revenues will rise by 9 percent. If costs rise by less than this, profits will rise.

7.6 Conclusion

An elasticity is the percentage change in one variable that is associated with a 1 percent change in another variable. Elasticities are simple, valuable tools managers can use to forecast sales and revenues. Elasticities allow managers to apply the results of sophisticated economic studies to their organizations.

Three elasticities are common: income elasticities, price elasticities, and cross-price elasticities. Income elasticities measure how much demand varies with income; price elasticities measure how much demand varies with the price of the product itself; and cross-price elasticities measure how much demand varies with the prices of complements and substitutes. Of these, price elasticity is the most important, because it guides pricing and contracting decisions.

Virtually all price elasticities of demand for healthcare products are negative, reflecting that higher prices generally reduce the quantity demanded. The overall demand for most healthcare products is inelastic, meaning a 1 percent increase in a product's price results in a reduction of less than 1 percent in the quantity sold. In most cases, though, the demand for an individual organization's products will be elastic, meaning a 1 percent increase in a product's price results in a reduction of more than 1 percent in the quantity sold. This difference is based on ease of substitution. There are few good substitutes for broadly defined healthcare products, so demand is inelastic. In contrast, the products of other healthcare providers are usually good substitutes for the products of a particular provider, so demand is elastic. When making decisions, managers must consider that their organization's products face elastic demands.

Homework

7.1 Why are elasticities useful for managers?

7.2 Why are price elasticities called "elastic" or "inelastic," when other elasticities are not?

7.3 Why is the demand for healthcare products usually inelastic?

7.4 Why is the demand for an individual firm's healthcare products usually elastic?

7.5 Average visits per week equal 640 when the copay is $40 and 360 when the copay is $60.

   a. Calculate the percentage change in visits, percentage change in price, and price elasticity of demand using 640 and $40 as the denominators for percentage change calculations.

   b. Calculate the percentage change in visits, percentage change in price, and price elasticity of demand using 360 and $60 as the denominators for percentage change calculations.

   c. Calculate the percentage change in visits, percentage change in price, and price elasticity of demand using 500 and $50 as the denominator for percentage change calculations. (This is an arc elasticity calculation.)

   d. How do your answers differ?

7.6 Sales are 3,100 at a price of $200 and 2,400 at a price of $300. Calculate the price elasticities of demand using $200 as the base value, then use $300 as the base value. Calculate the arc price elasticity and compare the three calculations. How do your answers differ?

7.7 Per capita income in Pitt County is $45,000. Per capita income in Chatham County is $38,000. Physician visits average 3.4 per year in Pitt County and 3.2 per year in Chatham County. What is the arc income elasticity of demand for visits?

7.8 Median household income in Clay County is $54,021. Median household income in Dent County is $28,739. In Clay County, 17.4 percent of residents smoke. In Dent County, 28.4 percent of residents smoke. What is the arc income elasticity of demand for tobacco use?

7.9 The price elasticity of demand is –1.2. Is demand elastic or inelastic?

7.10 The price elasticity of demand is –0.12. Is demand elastic or inelastic?

7.11 If the income elasticity of demand is 0.2, how would the volume of services change if income rose by 10 percent?

7.12 You are a manager for a regional health system. Using an estimate of the price elasticity of demand of –0.25, how much will ambulatory visits change if you raise prices by 5 percent?

7.13 If the cross-price elasticity of clinic visits with respect to pharmaceutical prices is –0.18, how much will ambulatory visits change if pharmacy prices rise by 5 percent? Are pharmaceuticals substitutes for or complements to clinic visits?

7.14 If the cross-price elasticity of clinic visits with respect to emergency department prices is 0.21, how much will ambulatory visits change if emergency department prices rise by 5 percent? Are emergency department visits substitutes for or complements to clinic visits?

7.15 If the income elasticity of demand is 0.03, how much will ambulatory visits change if incomes rise by 4 percent?

7.16 A study estimates that the price elasticity of demand for Effexor XR is –3.41, but the price elasticity of demand for tricyclic antidepressants as a whole is –0.22.
   a. Why is demand for Effexor XR more elastic than for antidepressants as a whole?
   b. What would happen to revenues if the makers of Effexor XR raised prices by 10 percent?
   c. What would happen to industry revenues if all manufacturers raised prices by 10 percent?
   d. Why are the answers so different? Does this make sense?

7.17 The price elasticity of demand for the services of Kim Jones, MD, is –4.0. The price elasticity of demand for physicians' services overall is –0.1.
   a. Why is demand so much more elastic for the services of Dr. Jones than for the services of physicians in general?
   b. If Dr. Jones reduced prices by 10 percent, how much would volume and revenue change?
   c. Suppose that all the physicians in the area reduced prices by 10 percent. How much would the total number of visits and revenue change?
   d. Why does it make sense that your answers to questions b and c are so different?

Chapter Glossary

Agency. An arrangement in which one person (the agent) takes actions on behalf of another (the principal)

Arc elasticity. An elasticity calculation that uses the average of the data to calculate percentage changes

Cross-price elasticity. The percentage change in the quantity demanded associated with a 1 percent change in the price of a related product

Elastic. A term used to describe demand when the quantity demanded falls
by more than 1 percent when the price rises by 1 percent. This term
is usually applied only to price elasticities of demand

Elasticity. The percentage change in a dependent variable associated with a
1 percent change in an independent variable

Income elasticity of demand. The percentage change in the quantity
demanded associated with a 1 percent increase in income

Inelastic. A term used to describe demand when the quantity demanded
falls by less than 1 percent when the price rises by 1 percent. This
term is usually applied only to price elasticities of demand

Price elasticity of demand. The percentage change in sales volume
associated with a 1 percent change in a product's price

References

Acton, J. P. 1975. "Nonmonetary Factors in the Demand for Medical Services:
Some Empirical Evidence." *Journal of Political Economy* 83: 595–614.

Anonymous. 1997. "Cut Wages and Increase Revenue by Reducing Wait Times."
Health Care Cost Reengineering Report 2 (5): 65–70.

Bush, S. H., M. R. Lao, K. L. Simmons, J. H. Goode, S. A. Cunningham, and B. C.
Calhoun. 2007. "Patient Access and Clinical Efficiency Improvement in a
Resident Hospital-based Women's Medicine Center Clinic." *American
Journal of Managed Care* 13 (12): 686–90.

Goldman, H. H., R. G. Frank, M. A. Burnam, H. A. Huskamp, M. S. Ridgely, S. L.
Normand, A. S. Young, C. L. Barry, V. Azzone, A. B. Busch, S. T. Azrin, G.
Moran, C. Lichtenstein, and M. Blasinsky. 2006. "Behavioral Health
Insurance Parity for Federal Employees." *New England Journal of Medicine*
354 (13): 1378–86.

Keeler, E., W. G. Manning, and K. B. Wells. 1988. "The Demand for Episodes of
Mental Health Services." *Journal of Health Economics* 7 (4): 369–92.

Lee, R. H., and J. Hadley. 1981. "Physicians' Fees and Public Medical Care
Programs." *Health Services Research* 16 (2): 185–203.

Manning, W. G., A. Leibowitz, M. S. Marquis, J. P. Newhouse, N. Duan, and E. B.
Keeler. 1987. "Health Insurance and the Demand for Medical Care:
Evidence from a Randomized Experiment." *American Economic Review* 77
(3): 251–77.

Newhouse, J. P., and C. E. Phelps. 1976. "New Estimates of Price and Income
Elasticities of Medical Care Services." In *The Role of Health Insurance in the
Health Services Sector*, edited by Richard Rosett. New York: Neal Watson.

Rosett, R. N., and L. Huang. 1973. "The Effect of Health Insurance on the
Demand for Medical Care." *Journal of Political Economy* 81: 281–305.

FORECASTING

Learning Objectives

After reading this chapter, students will be able to:

- **articulate** the importance of a good sales forecast,
- **describe** the attributes of a good sales forecast,
- **apply** demand theory to forecasts, and
- **use** simple forecasting tools appropriately.

Key Concepts

- Making and interpreting forecasts are important jobs for managers.
- Forecasts are planning tools, not rigid goals.
- Sales and revenue forecasts are applications of demand theory.
- Changes in demand conditions usually change forecasts.
- Good forecasts should be easy to understand, easy to modify, accurate, transparent, and precise.
- Forecasts combine history and judgment.
- Percentage adjustment, moving averages, and seasonalized regression analysis are common forecasting methods.
- Assessing external factors is vital to forecasting.

8.1 Introduction

Making and interpreting forecasts are important jobs for managers. Sales forecasts are especially important because many decisions hinge on what the organization expects to sell. Pricing decisions, staffing decisions, product launch decisions, and other crucial decisions are based on the organization's revenue and sales forecasts.

Inaccurate or misunderstood forecasts can hurt businesses. The organization can hire too many workers or too few. It can set prices too high or too low. It can add too much equipment or too little. At best, these sorts of forecasting problems will cut into profits; at worst, they may drive an organization out of business.

The consequences of bad or misapplied forecasts are particularly serious in healthcare. For example, underestimating the level of demand in the short term may result in stock shortages at a pharmacy or too few nurses on duty at a hospital. In both cases, the healthcare organization will suffer financially and, more important, put patients at risk. It will suffer because the costs of meeting unexpected demand are high and because the long-term consequences of failing to meet patients' needs are significant. The best outcome in this case will be unhappy patients; the worst outcome will be physicians who stop referring patients to the organization.

Overestimating sales can also have serious long-term effects. A hospital may add too many beds because its census forecast was too high. This surplus will depress profits for some time because the facility will have hired staff and added equipment to meet its overestimated forecast, and the costs of hiring and paying new employees and buying new equipment will substantially exceed actual sales profits. In extreme cases, bad forecasts may drive a firm out of business. A facility that borrows heavily in anticipation of higher sales that do not materialize may be unable to repay those debts. Bankruptcy may be the only option.

Sales and revenue forecasts are applications of demand theory. The factors that change sales and revenues also change demand. The most important influences on demand are the price of the product, rivals' prices for the product, prices for complements and substitutes, and demographics. Recognizing these influences can simplify forecasting considerably, as it focuses our attention on tracking what has changed.

8.2 What Is a Sales Forecast?

A sales forecast is a projection of the number of units (e.g., bed days, visits, doses) an organization expects to sell. The forecast must specify the time frame, marketing plan, and expected market conditions for which it is valid.

A forecast is a planning tool, not a rigid goal. Conditions may change. If they do, the organization's plan needs to be reassessed. Good management usually involves responding effectively to changes in the environment, not forging ahead as though nothing has shifted. In addition, fixed sales goals create incentives to behave opportunistically (that is, for employees to try to meet their goals instead of the organization's goals). For example, sales staff may harm the organization by making overblown claims to meet their goals, even though their actions will harm the company in the long run. Alternatively, sales managers may bid on unprofitable managed care contracts just to meet goals.

Whenever possible, a sales forecast should estimate the number of units expected to be sold, not revenues. The number of units to be sold

Case 8.1	**Building a New Urgent Care Center**

"It's a slam dunk," said Kim. "The volumes we've forecasted ensure that the new urgent care center will be profitable within six months."

"Great," replied Jordan, vice president of strategic management, "but I think it would be useful to walk through those numbers to put everyone at ease."

"OK, here's how we forecasted visits," said Kim. "There are 40,000 people living in our primary market area. National rates suggest that a population of this size will make 6,000 urgent care visits each year. Right now, our emergency department sees 2,500 urgent—but not emergent—visits each year. We believe that 1,500 of them will come to the urgent care center. Our seat-of-the-pants estimate is that Providence, the other hospital serving our primary market area, sees 2,000 urgent care patients per year in its emergency department. We expect to get half of those visits. We also expect that the added convenience of the urgent care center will bring in an additional 500 visits each year. So, 3,000 visits per year, each yielding revenue of $125, give us $375,000 in total revenue. We have fixed costs of $200,000. Our best estimate is that each visit has variable costs of $20, so we're talking profits of $115,000, for a margin on sales of 30 percent."

"That's nice and clear," said Jordan, "but I'd like to take a closer look. About half of the patients Providence sees would have to drive past Providence to get to our urgent care center. Do we have any indication that those folks will do that? My second concern is that our emergency department is open 24/7. The urgent care center will be open 82 hours per week. Can we really hope to capture 60 percent of the emergency department's urgent care patients?"

Discussion questions:

- What happens to profits if the urgent care center has only 2,000 visits?
- To what extent does Kim's forecast rely on judgment rather than data? Would additional information help resolve Jordan's concerns? What sort of data would you suggest gathering?
- Does building the urgent care center seem risky? Could you do anything to reduce the amount of risk?
- Would there be any advantages to planning for a small patient volume and letting your customers surprise you? Suppose you plan for 2,000 visits but volume turns out to be 3,000. What happens? Would underestimating be better or worse than planning for 3,000 and getting only 2,000?

determines staffing, materials, working capital, and other needs. In addition, costs often vary unevenly with volume. A small reduction in sales volume may save an entire shift's worth of wages (thereby avoiding considerable cost), or the cost incurred by an increase in sales may be insignificant if it requires no additional staff or equipment.

The dollar volume of sales can vary in response to factors that do not affect the resources needed to produce, market, or service sales. Discounts and price increases are examples of such factors. Revenues can vary even though neither volume nor costs change. Finally, managers can easily forecast revenue given a volume forecast. In general, managers should build their revenue estimates on sales volume estimates.

Good forecasts have five attributes. They should be

1. easy to understand,
2. easy to modify,
3. accurate (i.e., they contain the most probable actual values),
4. transparent about how variable they are, and
5. precise (i.e., they give the analyst as little wiggle room as possible).

These attributes often conflict. Managers may need to underplay how imprecise simple forecasts are because their audience is not prepared to consider variation. As Thompson (2002) points out, many decision makers are more comfortable working with a single, very precise estimate, even though it may be inaccurate. Precision and accuracy always conflict because a more precise forecast (80 to 85 visits per day) will always be less accurate than a less precise forecast (70 to 95 visits per day). Offering decision makers several precise scenarios is usually a good compromise. For example, busy decision makers generally can use a forecast such as: "Our baseline forecast is 82 visits per day for the next three months; our low forecast is 75 visits per day, and our high forecast is 89 visits per day."

8.3 Forecasting

All forecasts combine history and judgment. History is the only real source of data. For example, sales can be forecasted only on the basis of data on past sales of a product, past sales of similar products, past sales by rivals, or past sales in other markets. History is an imperfect guide to the future, but it is an essential starting point.

Judgment is also essential. It is the basis for deciding what data to use, how to use the data, and what statistical techniques, if any, to use. In many cases (such as introductions of new products or new competitive situations), managers who have insufficient data will have to base their forecasts mainly on judgment.

As mentioned in section 8.2, a forecast must specify the time frame, marketing plan, and expected market conditions for which it is valid. Changes in any of these factors will change the forecast.

A forecast applies to a given period. Extrapolating to a longer or shorter period is risky; conditions may change. The time frame varies according to the forecast's use. For example, a staffing plan may need a forecast for only the next few weeks. Additional staff can be hired over a longer time horizon. In contrast, budget plans usually need a forecast for the coming year. Organizations usually set their budgets a year in advance on the basis of projected sales. Strategic plans usually need a forecast for the next several years. Longer forecasts are generally less detailed and less reliable, but managers know to take these factors into account when they develop and use them.

Forecasts should be as short term as possible. A forecast for next month's sales will usually be more accurate than forecasts for the distant future, which are likely to be less accurate because important facts will have changed. Your competitors today are likely to be your competitors in a month. Your competitors in two years are likely to be different from your competitors today, so a forecast based on current market conditions will be poor.

Marketing plan changes will influence the forecast. A clinic that increases its advertising expects visits to increase. A forecast that does not consider this increase will usually be inaccurate. Increasing discounts to pharmacy benefits managers should result in increased sales for a pharmaceutical firm. Again, a forecast that does not account for additional discounts will usually be deficient. Any major changes in an organization's marketing efforts should change forecasts. If they do not, the organization should reassess the usefulness of its marketing initiatives.

Changes in market conditions also influence forecasts. For example, a major plant closing would probably reduce a local plastic surgeon's volume. Plant employees who had intended to undergo plastic surgery may opt to delay this elective procedure, and prospective patients who work for similar plants may defer discretionary spending in fear that they too may lose their jobs. Alternatively, a hospital closure will probably cause a competing hospital to forecast more inpatient days. Historical data have limited value in projecting such an effect if a similar closure has not occurred in the past. Approval of a new drug by the Food and Drug Administration should cause a pharmaceutical firm to forecast a decrease in sales for its competing product. This sort of change in market conditions is familiar, and the firm's marketing staff will probably draw on experience to predict the loss.

Analysts routinely use three forecasting methods: percentage adjustment, moving averages, and seasonalized regression analysis. If the data are adequate and the market has not changed too much, seasonalized regression analysis is the preferred method. However, whether the data are adequate and whether the market has changed too much are judgment calls.

Percentage adjustment increases or decreases the last period's sales volume by a percentage the analyst deems sensible. For example, if a hospital had an average daily census of 100 the previous quarter, and an analyst expects the census to fall an average of 1 percent per quarter, a reasonable forecast would be a census of 99. Because of its simplicity, managers often use percentage adjustment; however, this simplicity is also a shortcoming. In principle, a manager can use any percentage adjustment that he or she wants to. Without some requirement that percentage adjustments be well justified, this approach may not yield very accurate forecasts. For example a manager might justify a request for a new position based on a forecast that average daily census will increase by 5 percent, even though the average daily census had been falling for the last 14 quarters. In addition, percentage adjustment does not allow for seasonal effects. (*Seasonal effects* are systematic tendencies for particular days, weeks, months, or quarters to have above- or below-average volume.)

Demand theory can be used to add rigor to percentage adjustment. For example, if the price of a product has changed, an estimate of the percentage change in sales can be calculated by multiplying the percentage change in price by the price elasticity of demand. So, if an organization has chosen to raise prices by 3 percent and faces a price elasticity of demand of –4, sales will drop by 12 percent. Similar calculations can be used if the price of a substitute, the price of a complement, or consumer income has changed.

The moving-average method uses the average of data from recent periods to forecast sales. This method works well for short-term forecasts, although it tends to hide emerging trends and seasonal effects. Table 8.1 shows census data and a one-year moving average for Exemplar Hospital.

Table 8.1 also illustrates the calculation of a seasonalized regression format. Excel was used to estimate a regression model with a trend (a variable that increases in value as time passes) and three quarter indicators. The variable Q1 has a value of one if the data are from the first quarter; otherwise, its value is zero. Q2 equals one if the data are from the second quarter, and Q3 equals one if the data are from the third quarter. For technical reasons, the average response in the fourth quarter is represented by the constant. A negative regression coefficient for trend indicates that the census is in a downward trend. The results also show that the typical third-quarter census is smaller than average because the coefficient for Q3 is large, negative, and statistically significant.

The forecast based on seasonalized regression analysis is calculated as follows: $108.811 + (-0.334 \times 22) + 0.732$. Here, 108.811 is the estimate of the constant, –0.334 is the estimate of the trend coefficient, 22 is the quarter to which the forecast applies, and 0.732 is the estimate of the Q2 coefficient. Therefore, the seasonalized forecast is 102.2, slightly higher than the forecast based on the moving average. Overall the seasonalized forecast is a little more accurate than the one-year moving average. The mean absolute deviation for the regression is 2.3 for periods 5 through 21, and the mean absolute deviation for the moving average is 4.0.

Figure 8.1 shows an overview of the forecasting process. The main message of this figure is that a forecast is one part of the overall product

TABLE 8.1

Census Data for Exemplar Hospital

Quarter	Census	Moving Average	First	Second	Third	Trend
1	99		1	0	0	1
2	109		0	1	0	2
3	101		0	0	1	3
4	107		0	0	0	4
5	104	104.0	1	0	0	5
6	116	105.3	0	1	0	6
7	100	107.0	0	0	1	7
8	106	106.8	0	0	0	8
9	103	106.5	1	0	0	9
10	107	106.3	0	1	0	10
11	90	104.0	0	0	1	11
12	105	101.5	0	0	0	12
13	102	101.3	1	0	0	13
14	94	101.0	0	1	0	14
15	98	97.8	0	0	1	15
16	104	99.8	0	0	0	16
17	99	99.5	1	0	0	17
18	105	98.8	0	1	0	18
19	94	101.5	0	0	1	19
20	102	100.5	0	0	0	20
21	100	100.0	1	0	0	21
22		100.3				

Seasonalized Regression Model

	Coefficient	t-statistic	
Intercept	108.811	40.90	$R^2 = 0.55$
First quarter	−3.968	−1.53	$F_{(4,20)} = 4.98$
Second quarter	0.732	0.27	$p = 0.01$
Third quarter	−8.534	−3.16	
Trend	−0.334	−2.16	

management process. In addition, the forecast will change as managers' assessments of relevant internal factors (e.g., cost and quality), external factors (e.g., the competitive environment and reimbursement levels), and the marketing plan change.

FIGURE 8.1

An Overview of
the Forecasting
Process

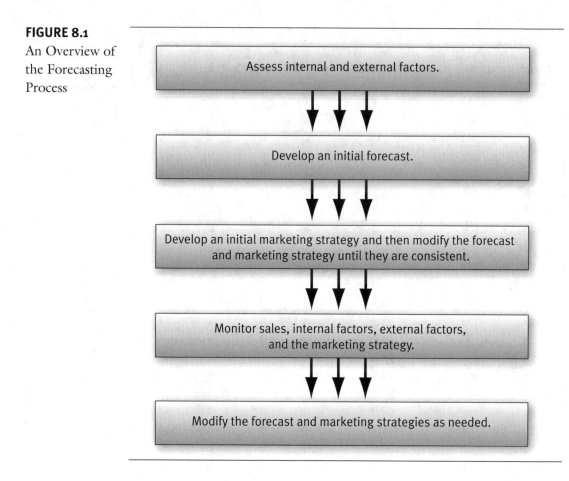

8.4 What Matters?

Assessment of external factors (i.e., factors beyond the organization's control) is vital to forecasting. General economic conditions are a prime example. Expected inflation and interest rates are good indicators of the state of the economy. Local market conditions, such as business rents and local wages, also play an important role.

Government actions also can have a major impact on healthcare firms. For example, changes in Medicare rates affect most healthcare firms. Alternatively, regulations can have a significant effect on costs. Expansion of Medicaid eligibility can have major effects on some hospitals and minor effects on others. Keep in mind that these sorts of changes will also affect most of your competitors, but forecasters would be ill-advised to ignore changes in government policy.

The plans of key competitors must also be considered. Closure of a competing clinic or hospital can increase volume significantly and quickly. Introduction of a generic drug can have a dramatic effect on a pharmaceutical

Sidebar 8.1 Simple Forecasting Techniques

A naïve forecast uses the value for the last period as the forecast for the next period—in other words, a 0 percent adjustment forecast.

	Sales	Naïve Forecast	Two-Period Moving Average
February	189		
March	217	189	
April	211	217	203
May	239	211	214
June	234	239	225
July	243	234	236.5

A moving-average forecast uses the average of the last n values. So, the first entry in the Two-Period Moving Average column is $(189 + 217) \div 2 = 203$.

To compare forecasting techniques, analysts sometimes use the mean absolute deviation, which is the average of the forecast's absolute deviations from the actual value. (When using the absolute deviation, it doesn't matter if a value is higher or lower than the actual; all the deviations are positive numbers.) For April through July the naïve forecast above has a mean absolute deviation of 12.0, and the two-period moving average has a mean absolute deviation of 12.1. From this perspective, the naïve forecast performs a little better.

These (and other) mechanistic forecasting methods do not allow managers to explore how changes in the environment are likely to affect sales. How would changes in insurance coverage change sales? Naïve forecasts and moving-average forecasts are little help in such situations.

manufacturer. Changes in competitors' pricing policies can have a major impact on sales.

Technological change is always an important issue. If a rival gains a technological advantage, your sales can drop sharply. For example, if a rival introduces minimally invasive coronary artery bypass graft surgery, admissions to your cardiac unit will probably drop significantly until you adopt similar technology. In other cases, your own advances may affect sales of substitute products. For example, introduction of highly reliable MRI may sharply reduce the demand for conventional colonoscopy. Keep in mind, however, that if you don't introduce technologies that add value for your customers, someone else will. A decision not to introduce an attractive product because it will cannibalize sales is usually a mistake.

Finally, although markets usually change slowly, differences in general market characteristics (e.g., median income and percentage with insurance coverage) may be important in forecasting sales of a new product.

Sidebar 8.2 Developing a Five-Year Forecast

Beech (2001) shows how to develop a five-year forecast for a hospital's strategic financial plan. He begins the analysis by defining the hospital's service area and then estimating how the population of the service area will change during the next five years in terms of gender and age. Next, Beech uses several data sources to forecast admission rates and length of stay for the services used by these population groups. (The hospital characterizes these services as medical and surgical, obstetrics and gynecology, pediatric, and psychiatric.) He then uses the hospital's own data and his estimates of overall admission rates and length of stay to calculate the hospital's market share for medical and surgical services, obstetric and gynecological services, pediatric services, and psychiatric services.

On the basis of these market share estimates, Beech develops four demand forecasts. His baseline forecast predicts that the hospital's market share and overall utilization will not change. His decreased utilization forecast predicts that overall days of care will drop by 10 percent but that the hospital will maintain its market share. His decreased market share forecast predicts that the hospital's market share will fall by 2 percent, and his increased market share forecast predicts that the hospital's market share will rise by 2 percent. (The decreased market share and increased market share forecasts predict that utilization rates will not change.) History suggests that Beech's decreased utilization forecast is most likely to occur. To the relief of the hospital's management, the area's population growth will offset most of the drop in days of care per thousand residents, so overall days of care will drop by less than 1 percent. However, this scenario implies that pediatric days will drop by more than 7 percent, so the hospital will need to look carefully at costs in this service line.

Assessment of internal factors (i.e., factors within an organization's control) is also vital to forecasting. For example, existing production may limit sales, or may have in the past. If so, changes in capacity or productivity need to be considered. Changes in the availability of resources and personnel can also have a powerful effect on sales. For many healthcare organizations, the entry or exit of a key physician can dramatically shape volume. In addition, changes in the size, support, composition, and organization of the sales staff can affect sales dramatically. For instance, a small drug firm may experience a large increase in sales if one of its products is marketed by a larger firm's sales staff.

Failures or improvements in key systems can also have dramatic effects on sales. Breakdowns in its phone or scheduling system may drive away a clinic's potential customers. Fixing the phone system, in contrast, might be the most effective marketing campaign the clinic ever launched.

| Case 8.2 | **Forecasting the Demand for Transfusions** |

"Our blood inventories are shrinking," said Dr. Allen, "and I'm worried that we might not be able to supply our customers if there's a surge in demand. We need to do something. And it needs to be smart, because the shelf life of blood is only six weeks. Simply collecting more may not solve our problem."

At this point, Kim chimed in, "We need to do more than just predict our annual volume. We need a monthly forecast. That way we can target our drives so that we collect enough blood shortly before we expect to use it. Less blood will expire, and we will only need to address unexpected spikes in use."

"The good news," said Taylor, "is that we have monthly data for the last six years. We should be able to use them. I know that Dr. Pereira (2004) tested a number of time-series models and suggested several that work reasonably well. I think he found some clear seasonal effects."

Discussion questions:

- What sort of model would you recommend to predict the demand for blood? What would you do with your predictions?
- Why would the presence of seasonal effects be important?
- Taylor suggested using a statistical model to forecast demand. What judgment does a statistical model require?
- What sorts of changes in the environment would you need to account for in your forecasting model?

8.5 Conclusion

Making and interpreting forecasts are important tasks for healthcare managers. Not only are most crucial decisions based on sales forecasts but also the consequences of overestimating or underestimating demand can be catastrophic. Overestimating demand can put the financial future of an organization at risk, and underestimating demand can compromise the care of patients and harm the organization's reputation.

Analysts should apply demand theory to their sales forecasts to better recognize changes. Demand theory limits what analysts need to consider: the price of the product, the price of substitutes, and the price of complements. The key idea of demand theory is that the out-of-pocket price is what drives most consumer demand. The amount the consumer has to pay depends largely on the terms of his or her insurance contract. Is the product covered? What is the required copayment? Changes in the answers to these two questions can shift sales sharply. The same concerns affect the prices of substitutes. The most important substitutes are similar products offered by rivals, but other products that meet some of the same needs should also be considered.

Demographic factors are important. Population size, income per capita, the age distribution of the population, the ethnic makeup of the population, and the insurance coverage of the population are some examples. Although vital, demographic factors tend to be stable in the short term. Demographics are much more important in long-range forecasts.

An old joke notes that "Forecasting is hard, especially when it involves the future." The joke reveals a core truth about forecasting: you often will be wrong. Knowing that, a shrewd manager will make decisions that can be modified as conditions change. That shrewd manager will also know which data are likely to be the most problematic or most variable and will monitor those data carefully.

Management decisions require sales forecasts. Off-the-cuff forecasts often fail to consider key factors and lead to risky decisions. Imperfect forecasts can be used to make decisions as long as you recognize that your predictions will sometimes be wrong and structure your decisions accordingly.

Homework

	Clinic 1	Clinic 2	Clinic 3	Clinic 4	Total
This year	16,640	41,600	24,960	33,280	116,480
Next year	?	?	?	?	121,139

8.1   The table lists visits for each of the four clinics operated by your system. You anticipate that volumes will increase by 4 percent next year. Forecast visits for each clinic, and explain what assumptions underlie your forecasts. For example, are you sure that all of the clinics can serve additional clients?

8.2   Your data suggest that Clinic 2 is operating at capacity and highly efficient. Its output is unlikely to increase. Furthermore, Clinic 4 has unused capacity but is unlikely to attract additional patients. How would these facts change your answer to question 1? Continue to assume that overall volume will rise to 121,139.

8.3   You estimate that the price elasticity of demand for clinic visits is –0.25. You anticipate that a major insurer will increase the copayment from $20 to $25. This insurer covers 40,000 of your patients, and those patients average 2.5 visits per year. What is your forecast of the change in the number of visits?

8.4   A major employer has just added health insurance coverage for its employees. Consequently, 5,000 of your patients will pay a $30 copayment rather than the list price of $100 per visit. These patients average 2.2 visits per year. You believe the price elasticity of demand is between –0.15 and –0.35. What is your forecast of the change in the number of visits?

8.5 The table below shows data on asthma-related visits. Is there evidence that these visits vary by quarter? Can you detect a trend? A powerful test would be to run a multiple regression in Excel. If the function is already loaded, you will find it in Tools > Data Analysis > Regression. If not, go to Tools > Add-ins > Analysis Tool Pak to load it. To test for quarterly differences, create a variable called Quarter 1 that equals 1 if the data are for the first quarter and 0 otherwise; a variable called Quarter 2 that equals 1 if the data are for the second quarter and 0 otherwise; and a variable called Quarter 4 that equals 1 if the data are for the fourth quarter and 0 otherwise. (Because you will accept the default, which is to have constant term in your regression equation, do not include an indicator variable for Quarter 3.) Also create a variable called Trend that increases by 1 each quarter.

	Q1	Q2	Q3	Q4
2001			1,513	1,060
2002	1,431	1,123	994	679
2003	1,485	886	1,256	975
2004	1,256	1,156	1,163	1,062
2005	1,200	1,072	1,563	531
2006	1,022	1,169		

8.6 Your marketing department estimates that Medicare urology visits = 5 – (1.0 × C) + (–6.5 × T_O) + (5 × T_R) + (0.01 × Y). Here, C denotes the Medicare copayment (now $20); TO is waiting time in your clinic (now 30 minutes); T_R is waiting time in your competitor's clinic (now 40 minutes); and Y is per capita income (now $40,000).
   a. How many visits do you anticipate?
   b. Medicare's allowed fee is $120. What revenue do you anticipate?
   c. What might change your forecast of visits and revenue?

8.7 Because of fluctuations in insurance coverage, the average price paid out of pocket by an urgent care center varied. The number of visits per month also varied, and an analyst believes the two are related. The analyst also thinks there is a trend. Run a regression of Q on P and Period to test these hypotheses. Then use the estimated parameters a, b, and c and the values of Period and P to predict Q (sales). The prediction equation is: Q = a + (b × Period) + (c × P).

Period	1	2	3	4	5	6	7	8	9	10	11	12
P	$21	$18	$15	$24	$18	$21	$18	$15	$20	$19	$24	$20
Q	193	197	256	179	231	214	247	273	223	225	198	211

8.8   Using the data in question 8.7:

   a.   Calculate the naïve estimator, which is $Q_t = Q_{t-1}$.

   b.   Calculate the two-period moving-average forecast.

   c.   Calculate the mean absolute deviation for the regression forecast, the naïve forecast, and the two-period moving-average forecast.

   d.   Which forecast seems to perform the best? Why?

8.9   Sales data are displayed below.

   a.   Calculate the naïve estimator, which is $Sales_t = Sales_{t-1}$.

   b.   Calculate the two-period and three-period moving averages.

   c.   Calculate the mean absolute deviation for each of the forecasting methods.

Month	Sales	Month	Sales
February	224	January	260
March	217	February	284
April	211	March	280
May	239	April	271
June	234	May	302
July	243	June	286
August	238	July	297
September	243	August	301
October	251	September	309
November	259	October	314
December	270		

8.10 A pharmaceutical company produces a sinus medicine. Monthly sales (in thousands of doses) for the past three years are shown in the following table:

Jan	Feb	Mar	Apr	May	June	July	Aug	Sept	Oct	Nov	Dec
6,788	8,020	1,848	410	586	2,260	2,232	8,018	9,384	6,916	5,698	6,940
9,136	7,420	3,350	1,998	1,972	3,572	4,506	10,474	13,358	8,232	8,218	10,248
9,628	7,826	3,528	2,126	2,070	3,762	4,754	11,010	14,040	8,646	8,634	10,782

   a.   Develop a regression model that allows for trend and seasonal components. Obtain the Excel output for this model.

   b.   Calculate a two-period moving-average forecast.

   c.   Compare the mean absolute deviations for these approaches.

   d.   Use one of these models to forecast sales for each month of year 3.

Chapter Glossary

Exponential moving average. An average that gives decreasing weight to older data. For example, a common formula is $\hat{x}_t = \alpha \hat{x}_{t-1} + (1 - \alpha)x_{t-1}$, which gives less and less weight over time to the observations that produced $\hat{x}_{t-1}$

Mean absolute deviation. The average absolute difference between a forecast and the actual value. It is absolute because it converts both 9 and –9 to 9. The Excel function = abs( ) performs this conversion

Moving average. The unweighted mean of the previous n data points

Percentage adjustment. Percentage adjustment of the past n periods of historic demand. (The adjustment is essentially a best guess of what is expected to happen in the next year.)

Seasonalized regression analysis. A least squares regression that includes variables that identify subperiods (e.g., weeks) that historically have had above- or below-trend sales

References

Beech, A. J. 2001. "Market-based Demand Forecasting Promotes Informed Strategic Financial Planning." *Healthcare Financial Management* 55 (11): 46–56.

Pereira, A. 2004. "Performance of Time-Series Methods in Forecasting the Demand for Red Blood Cell Transfusion." *Transfusion* 44 (5): 739–46.

Thompson, K. M. 2002. "Variability and Uncertainty Meet Risk Management and Risk Communication." *Risk Analysis* 22 (3): 647–54.

SUPPLY AND DEMAND ANALYSIS

After reading this chapter, students will be able to:

- **define** demand and supply curves,
- **interpret** demand and supply curves,
- **use** demand and supply analysis to make simple forecasts, and
- **identify** factors that shift demand and supply curves.

- A *supply curve* describes how much producers are willing to sell at different prices.
- A *demand curve* describes how much consumers are willing to buy at different prices.
- A demand curve describes how much consumers are willing to pay at different levels of output.
- At the *equilibrium price*, producers want to sell the amount that consumers want to buy.
- Markets generally move toward equilibrium outcomes.
- Expansion of insurance usually makes the equilibrium price and quantity rise.
- Insurance and professional advice influence the demand for medical goods and services.
- Regulation and technology influence the supply of medical goods and services.
- Demand and supply curves shift when a factor other than the product price changes.

9.1 Introduction

Healthcare markets are in a constant state of flux. Prices rise and fall. Volumes rise and fall. New products succeed at first and then fall by the wayside.

Familiar products falter and revive. Economics teaches us that, underneath the seemingly random fluctuations of healthcare markets, systematic patterns can be detected. Understanding these systematic patterns requires an understanding of supply and demand. Even though healthcare managers need to focus on the details of day-to-day operations, they also need an appreciation of the overview that supply and demand analysis can give them.

The basics of supply and demand illustrate the usefulness of economics. Even with little data, managers can forecast the effects of changes in policy or demographics using a supply and demand analysis. For example, the impact of added taxes on hospitals' prices, the impact of increased insurance coverage on the output mix of physicians, and the impact of higher electricity prices on pharmacies' prices can be analyzed. Supply and demand analysis is a powerful tool that managers can use to make broad strategic decisions or detailed pricing decisions.

9.1.1 Supply Curves

Figure 9.1 is a basic supply and demand diagram. The vertical axis shows the price of the good or service. In this simple case, the price sellers receive is the same price buyers pay. (Insurance and taxes complicate matters, as the price the buyer pays is different from the price the seller receives.) The horizontal axis shows the quantity customers bought and producers sold.

The supply curve (labeled S) describes how much producers are willing to sell at different prices. From another perspective, it describes what the price must be to induce producers to be willing to sell different quantities. The supply curve in Figure 9.1 slopes up, as do most supply curves. This upward slope means that, when the price is higher, producers are willing to sell *more of a good or service*, or *more producers* are willing to sell a good or service. When the price is higher, producers are more willing to add workers, equipment, and other resources to sell more. In addition, higher prices allow firms to enter a market they could not enter at lower prices. When prices are low, only the most efficient firms can profitably participate in a market. But when prices are higher, firms with higher costs can also earn acceptable profits.

9.1.2 Demand Curves

The demand curve (labeled D) describes how much consumers are willing to buy at different prices. From another perspective, it describes how much the marginal consumer (the one who would not make a purchase at a higher price) is willing to pay at different levels of output. The demand curve in Figure 9.1 slopes down, meaning that, to sell more of a product, its price must be cut. Such a sales increase might be the result of an increase in the share of the population that buys a good or service, an increase in consumption per purchaser, or some mix of the two.

FIGURE 9.1
Equilibrium

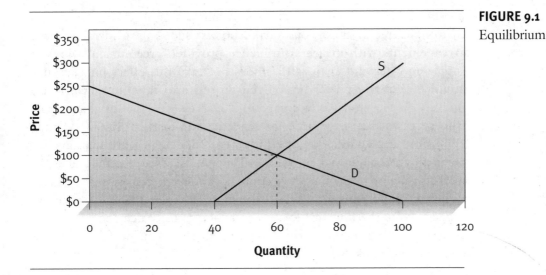

9.1.3 Equilibrium

The demand and supply curves intersect at the equilibrium price and quantity. At the equilibrium price, the amount producers want to sell equals the amount consumers want to buy. In Figure 9.1, consumers want to buy 60 units and producers want to sell 60 units when the price is $100.

Markets tend to move toward equilibrium points. If the price is above the equilibrium price, producers' sales forecasts will not be met. Sometimes producers cut prices to sell more. Sometimes producers cut production. Either strategy tends to equate supply and demand. Alternatively, if the price is below the equilibrium price, consumers will quickly buy up the available stock. To meet this shortage, producers may raise prices or produce more. Either strategy tends to equate supply and demand.

Markets will not always be in equilibrium, especially if conditions change quickly, but the incentive to move toward equilibrium is strong. Producers typically can change prices faster than they can increase or decrease production. A high price today does not mean a high price tomorrow. Prices are likely to fall as additional capacity becomes available. Likewise, a low price today does not mean a low price tomorrow. Prices are likely to rise as capacity decreases. We will explore this concept in more detail in our examination of the effects of managed care on the incomes of primary care physicians.

9.1.4 Professional Advice and Imperfect Competition

We offer two notes of caution. Healthcare markets are complex. The influence of professional advice on consumer choices is a complication of particular concern. The assumption that changes in supply will affect consumers' choices (i.e., demand) can be misleading. If changes in factors that ought not to affect consumers' choices (such as providers' financial arrangements with insurers) influence providers' recommendations, a supply and demand analysis that does not take this effect into account could be equally misleading. Even more important, few healthcare markets fit the model of a competitive market (i.e., lots of competitors who perceive they have little influence on the market price). We must condition any analysis on the judgment that healthcare markets are competitive enough that conventional supply curves are useful guides. In markets that are not competitive enough, producers' responses to changes in market conditions are likely to be more complex than supply curves suggest. Note that this text focuses on applications of demand and supply analysis in which neither providers' influence on demand nor imperfect competition are likely to be problems.

9.2 Demand and Supply Shifts

We term a movement along a demand curve a *change in the quantity demanded*. In other words, a movement along a demand curve traces the link between the price consumers are willing to pay and the quantity they demand. Demand and supply analysis is most useful, however, in understanding how the equilibrium price and quantity will change in response to shifts in demand or supply. This application helps managers the most. With limited information, a working manager can sketch the impact of a change in policy on the markets of most concern.

What factors might cause the demand curve to shift to the right (greater demand at every price or higher prices for every quantity)? We need detailed empirical work to verify the responses of demand to market conditions, but the standard list is short. Typically, a shift to the right results from an increase in income, an increase in the price of a substitute (a good or service used instead of the product in question), a decrease in the price of a complement (a good or service used along with the product in question), or a change in tastes.

Economists often use mathematical notation to describe demand. $Q = D(P,Y)$ is an example of this notation. It says that the quantity demanded varies with prices (represented by P) and income (represented by Y), which means that quantity, the relevant prices, and income are systematically related. A demand curve traces this relationship when income and all prices other than the price of the product itself do not change.

What factors might cause the supply curve to shift to the right (greater supply at every price or lower prices at every quantity)? Typically, a shift to the right results from a reduction in the price of an input, an

Case 9.1   **Worrying About Demand Shifts**

"You know, this business is changing," said Kim. "It used to be that an administrator like me had to worry only about running a good nursing home and keeping an eye on the other nursing homes in town, but these days we have more competitors than I can shake a stick at. Some of the folks at Sunshine Assisted Living would have been residents in our nursing home a few years ago. Not today, though. We admit their residents only when they are getting close to needing total care. Without changing offices, I feel like I switched from running a nursing home to running a hospice. The thing that has me spooked, though, is this new home health agency. It has billboards out on the interstate with a picture of a senior citizen and a slogan that says, 'Stay healthy. Stay Active. Stay home.' I'm worried that it will siphon off a significant part of our residents. It's just supply and demand."

With that Kim jumped up, went over to the whiteboard, and drew a simple graph (Figure 9.2). "Here's where we are today. We have a census of about 150, and we're doing fine. But when those home health folks are done with us, we'll be lucky to have a census of 100. I'm worried."

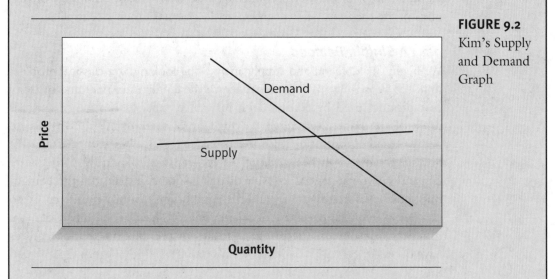

FIGURE 9.2
Kim's Supply and Demand Graph

"Whoa, partner," interrupted Kelly, who handles marketing. "I like the graph, but I don't think a home health agency is going to have that sort of impact on us. A 2007 study out of Brown University by Andrea Gruneir and her colleagues did not find the sorts of impacts you are describing. I just don't think many of our residents are candidates for home health services. By the time we see them, they need more care than most home health agencies can offer."

(continued)

Case 9.1 continued

Discussion questions:

- Figure 9.2 shows the current situation. What did Kim think the graph would look like after the home health care agency entered the market? What did Kelly think the new graph would look like?
- Over the next few years, what sorts of demographic changes seem likely to shift the demand for nursing home care?
- What sorts of changes in the local market might cause the sort of shift in demand that Kim is concerned about?

improvement in technology, or an easing of regulations. In mathematical notation, we can describe supply as $Q = S(P,W)$. Here, W represents the prices of inputs (the factors like labor, land, equipment, buildings, and supplies that a business uses to produce its product). Unless technology or regulations are the focus of an analysis, we do not make their role explicit.

9.2.1 A Shift in Demand

We begin our demand and supply analyses by looking at a classical problem in health economics: What will happen to the equilibrium price and quantity of a product used by consumers if insurance expands? Insurance expands when the insurance plan agrees to pay a larger share of the bill or the proportion of the population with insurance increases. This sort of change in insurance causes a *shift in demand*. As you can see in Figure 9.3, the entire demand curve rotates. As a result of this insurance expansion, the equilibrium price rises from P_1 to P_2 and the equilibrium quantity rises from Q_1 to Q_2. For example, as coverage for pharmaceuticals has become a part of more Americans' insurance, the prices and sales of prescription pharmaceuticals have risen.

9.2.2 A Shift in Supply

Figure 9.4 depicts a shift in supply. The supply curve has contracted from S_1 to S_2. This shift means that at every price, producers want to supply a smaller volume. Alternatively, it means that to produce each volume, producers require a higher price. A change in regulations might result in a shift like the one from S_1 to S_2. For example, suppose that state regulations mandated improved care planning and record keeping for nursing homes. Some nursing homes might close down, but the majority would raise prices for private-pay patients to cover the increased cost of care. The net effect would be an increase in the equilibrium price from P_1 to P_2 and a reduction in the

Sidebar 9.1 The Supply of Physicians' Services

Empirical analyses of supply usually find that an increase in earnings results in higher volume (i.e., supply curves usually slope up). A study described by Rizzo and Blumenthal (1994) found that young, male, self-employed physicians fit this pattern. A 1 percent increase in hourly earnings increased annual practice hours by 0.23 percent. One reason why the response was so muted is that an increase in hourly earnings also increases total income, and having a higher income usually leads to a reduction in hours. Confirming this supposition, the study found that a 1 percent increase in income from all sources reduced annual hours by 0.26 percent. Many young physicians have spouses with high earning potential, which also tends to reduce hours. A 1 percent increase in a physician's spouse's income reduced annual hours by 0.02 percent. In other words, the study found that change in either nonpractice income or in a spouse's earnings shifts the supply curve. So, both practice and nonpractice earnings affected annual hours of work. As is usually the case in labor supply analyses, both effects were relatively inelastic.

The implication for managers is that the way to get people to supply what you want is to pay them. Paying for visits will increase visits. Paying for quality will increase quality. This maxim appears to apply to high-income and low-income workers alike.

equilibrium quantity from Q_1 to Q_2. A manager should be able to forecast this effect with no information other than the realization that the demand for nursing home care is relatively inelastic (meaning that the slope of the demand curve is steep) and that the regulation would shift the supply curve inward.

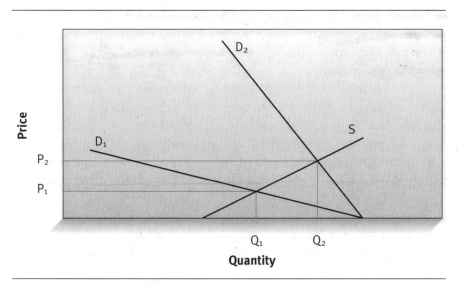

FIGURE 9.3

An Expansion of Insurance

FIGURE 9.4
A Supply Shift

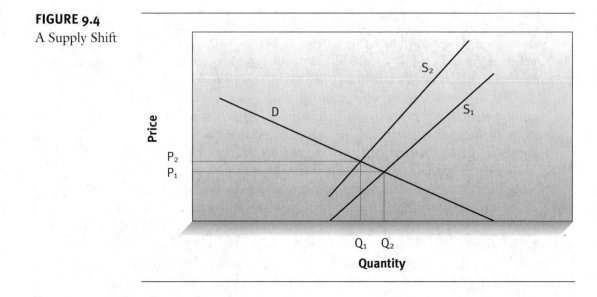

Note that responses to changing market conditions depend on how much time passes. A change in technology, such as the development of a new surgical technique, initially will have little effect on supply. Over time, however, as more surgeons become familiar with the technique, its impact on supply will grow. Short-term supply and demand curves generally look different from long-term supply and demand curves. The more time consumers and producers have to respond, the more their behavior changes.

9.3 Shortage and Surplus

A *shortage* exists when the quantity demanded at the prevailing price exceeds the quantity supplied. In markets that are free to adjust, the price should rise so that equilibrium is restored. At a higher price, less will be demanded, leaving a greater supply.

In some markets, though, prices cannot adjust, often because a public or private insurer sets prices too low and consumers demand more than producers are willing to supply. Figure 9.5 depicts a shortage situation. The equilibrium price is P* and the equilibrium quantity is Q*, but the insurer has set a price of P_2, so consumers demand Q_D and producers supply Q_S. Because the price cannot adjust, there is a shortage equal to $Q_D - Q_S$.

A *surplus* exists when the quantity supplied at the prevailing price exceeds the quantity demanded. In markets that are free to adjust, the price should fall so that equilibrium is restored. In some markets, prices are free to

Sidebar 9.2 Did California Have a Shortage of Dental Hygienists?

In the 1990s, dentists in California believed there was a shortage of dental hygienists. A team from the University of California examined the evidence to see if this was true (Brown, Finlayson, and Scheffler 2007). The researchers focused on whether wages for dental hygienists increased—the best test for determining the presence of a surplus. They found that inflation-adjusted wages rose by 48 percent between 1999 and 2002, indicating there was a shortage. Between 2002 and 2005, however, inflation-adjusted wages did not change, which suggested a new equilibrium had been reached.

The shortage of dental hygienists likely resulted from a fairly rapid increase in demand for dental services during the 1990s. An increase in the number of people with dental insurance, increased incomes, and an increased over-55 population were likely contributors to this expansion of demand.

The shortage appears to have eased as inactive hygienists returned to the workforce and as dentists reduced their hiring plans in response to higher wages. The overall number of hygienists did not appreciably change.

fall but do so slowly. For example, in the 1990s, many hospitals had unfilled hospital beds because the combination of managed care and new technology reduced the demand for inpatient care. Over time, insurance companies used this excess capacity to secure much lower rates (even though Medicare and Medicaid rates remained unchanged), and enough hospitals closed or downsized to eliminate the excess capacity.

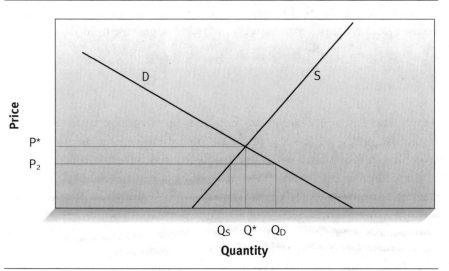

FIGURE 9.5

A Shortage

FIGURE 9.6
Higher RN
Wages Shift
Demand for
LPNs

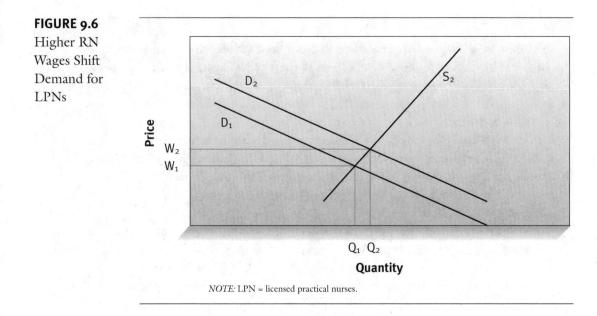

NOTE: LPN = licensed practical nurses.

9.4 Analyses of Multiple Markets

Demand and supply models can also be helpful in forecasting the effects of shifts in one market on the equilibrium in another. Such forecasts can be made only if the markets are related—that is, the products need to be complements or substitutes.

Spetz and colleagues (2006) provided an example of this effect. They showed that the demand for licensed practical nurses increased as the wages of registered nurses rose (as a result of the shortage of registered nurses [RNs]) (see Figure 9.6). Increases in the wages of registered nurses shifted the demand curve for licensed practical nurses from D_1 to D_2. As a result, employment of licensed practical nurses rose from Q_1 to Q_2 and wages rose from W_1 to W_2.

9.5 Conclusion

Supply and demand analysis can help managers anticipate the effects of changes in policy, technology, or prices. Supply and demand analysis is most valuable as a tool managers can use to quickly anticipate the effects of shifts in demand or supply curves. Short-term shifts in demand are likely to result from one of two factors: changes in insurance or shifts in the prices or characteristics of substitutes or complements. Short-term shifts in supply are likely to result from one of three factors: changes in regulations, shifts in the prices or characteristics of inputs, or changes in technology.

Make sure you understand the basic shapes of demand and supply curves. Most demand curves slope down, which means consumers will buy

---

Case 9.2	**What Will Happen to the Incomes of Pediatricians?**

In the early 1990s, concerns about the supply of pediatricians led to an expansion of pediatric training. As a result, the number of pediatricians is expected to grow from about 45,000 in 2005 to about 60,000 in 2020. In contrast, the number of children is expected to grow by less than 10 percent, meaning that the number of children per pediatrician should fall by about 20 percent (Shipman, Lurie, and Goodman 2004).

The decline in the number of children per pediatrician seems likely to result in lower incomes for pediatricians. Further, this decrease may be amplified by the emergence of retail clinics that are staffed by nurse practitioners and offer convenient, walk-in services for many common childhood illnesses.

Discussion questions:

- Model the effects of the drop in the number of children per pediatrician using per pediatrician demand and supply curves. How do you expect those curves to shift over time? What impact will this shift have on the incomes of pediatricians?
- If retail clinics continue to expand, how will they affect the market for pediatricians' services?
- Many children are uninsured. How would a program that provided coverage for all children affect your conclusions?
- If the incomes of pediatricians started dropping, would you expect the number of pediatricians to continue to grow?

---

more if prices are lower. It also means that consumers who are willing to purchase a product only at a low price do not place a high value on it. In contrast, most supply curves slope up, which means higher prices will motivate producers to sell additional output (or motivate more producers to sell the same output).

Homework

9.1 Physicians' offices supply some urgent care services (i.e., services patients seek for prompt attention but not for preservation of life or limb).
   a. Name three other providers of urgent care services.
   b. What sort of shift in supply or demand would result in a market equilibrium with higher prices and sales volume?
   c. What might cause such a shift?
   d. What sort of shift in supply or demand would result in a market equilibrium with higher prices but lower sales volume?
   e. What might cause such a shift?

9.2 Suppose the market equilibrium for immunizations is $40 and the
volume is 25,000.
   a. Identify three providers of immunization services.
   b. What sort of shift in supply or demand would reduce both prices
       and sales volume?
   c. What might cause such a shift?
   d. What sort of shift in supply or demand would result in a market
       equilibrium with a price above $40 and a volume below 25,000?
   e. What might cause such a shift?

9.3 The table at right contains data
on the number of doses of an
antihistamine sold per month in
a small town.

Price	Demand	Supply
$10	185	208
$9	187	205
$8	188	202
$7	190	199
$6	191	196
$5	193	193
$4	194	190
$3	196	187
$2	197	184
$1	199	181

   a. To sell 196 doses to
       customers, what will the
       price need to be?
   b. For stores to be willing to
       sell 196 doses, what will the
       price need to be?
   c. How many doses will
       customers want to buy if the price is $2?
   d. How many doses will suppliers want to sell if the price is $2?
   e. Is there excess supply or excess demand at $2?
   f. What is the equilibrium price? How can you tell?

9.4 The table at right contains demand
and supply data for eyeglasses in a
local market.

Price	Demand	Supply
$300	7,400	8,320
$290	7,480	8,200
$280	7,520	8,080
$270	7,600	7,960
$260	7,640	7,840
$250	7,720	7,720
$240	7,760	7,600
$230	7,840	7,480
$220	7,880	7,360

   a. At $280, how many pairs will
       consumers want to buy?
   b. How many pairs will consumers
       want to buy if the price is $290?
   c. How many pairs will stores want
       to sell at $290?
   d. Is $290 the equilibrium price?
   e. Is there excess supply or excess demand at $290?
   f. What is the equilibrium price? How can you tell?

9.5 Below is a basic demand and supply graph for home care services.
Identify the equilibrium price and quantity. Label them P* and Q*.
   a. Retirements drive up the wages of home care workers. How would
       the graph change? How would P* and Q* change?
   b. Improved technology lets home care workers monitor use of
       medications without going to clients' homes. How would the
       graph change? How would P* and Q* change?

c. The number of people needing home care services increases. How would the graph change? How would P* and Q* change?

d. A change in Medicare rules expands coverage for home care services. How would the graph change? How would P* and Q* change?

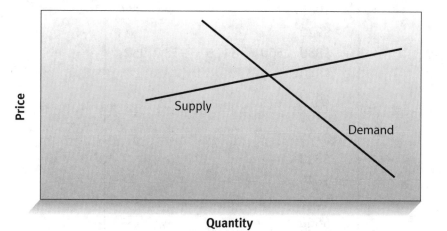

9.6 The demand function is Q = 600 – P, with P being the price paid by consumers. Put a list of prices ranging from $400 to $0 in a column labeled P. (Use intervals of $50.)

a. Consumers have insurance with 40 percent coinsurance. For each price, calculate the amount that consumers pay. (Put this figure in column P$_{Net}$.)

b. Calculate the quantity demanded when there is insurance. (Put this figure in column D$_I$.)

c. Plot the demand curve, putting P (not P$_{Net}$) on the vertical axis.

d. The quantity supplied equals 2 × P. Put these values in a column labeled S.

e. What is the equilibrium price?

f. How much do consumers spend?

g. How much does the insurer spend?

9.7 The demand function is Q = 1,000 – (0.5 × P). P is the price paid by consumers. Calculate the quantity demanded when there is no insurance. (Put these values in column D$_U$ on the table below.)

a. The state mandates coverage with 20 percent coinsurance, meaning the demand function becomes 1,000 – (0.5 × 0.2 × P).

b. For each price, calculate the amount consumers pay. (Put this figure in column P$_{Net}$.)

c. Calculate the quantity demanded when there is insurance. (Put this figure in column D$_I$.)

d. Plot the two demand curves, putting P (not P$_{Net}$) on the vertical axis.

e. How do D_U and D_I differ? Which is more elastic?

P	D_U	P_{Net}	D_I	S
$1,000				
$960				
$920				
$880	560	$176	912	952
$840				
$800				
$760				
$720				
$680				
$640				
$600				
$560				

9.8   The supply function for the product in question 9.7 is 160 + (0.9 × P). P is the price received by the seller. At the equilibrium price, the quantity demanded will equal the quantity supplied.
   a. What was the equilibrium price before coverage? After?
   b. After coverage begins, how much will the tests cost insurers? How much will the tests cost patients? How much did patients pay for tests before coverage started?

9.9   Consumers who can buy health insurance through an employer get a tax subsidy. Use demand and supply analysis to assess how this affects consumers who cannot buy insurance through an employer.

9.10 Why are price controls unlikely to make consumers better off if a market is reasonably competitive?

9.11 Make the business case why healthcare providers should advocate for expansion of insurance coverage for the poor.

Chapter Glossary

Demand curve. Curve that describes how much consumers are willing to buy at different prices

Demand shift. Shift that occurs when a factor other than price of the product (e.g., consumer incomes) changes

Equilibrium price. Price at which the quantity demanded equals the quantity supplied (There is no shortage or surplus.)

Shortage. Situation in which the quantity demanded at the prevailing price exceeds the quantity supplied

Supply curve. Curve that describes how much producers are willing to sell at different prices

Supply shift. Shift that occurs when a factor (e.g., an input price) other than price of the product changes

References

Brown, T., T. L. Finlayson, and R. M. Scheffler. 2007. "How Do We Measure Shortages of Dental Hygienists and Dental Assistants? Evidence from California: 1997–2005." *Journal of the American Dental Association* 138 (1): 94–100.

Gruneir, A., K. L. Lapane, S. C. Miller, and V. Mor. 2007. "Long-term Care Market Competition and Nursing Home Dementia Special Care Units." *Medical Care* 45 (8): 739–45.

Rizzo, J. A., and D. Blumenthal. 1994. "Physician Labor Supply: Do Income Effects Matter?" *Journal of Health Economics* 13 (4): 433–53.

Shipman, S. A., J. D. Lurie, and D. C. Goodman. 2004. "The General Pediatrician: Projecting Future Workforce Supply and Requirements." *Pediatrics* 113 (3): 435–42.

Spetz, J., W. T. Dyer, S. Chapman, and J. A. Seago. 2006. "Hospital Demand for Licensed Practical Nurses." *Western Journal of Nursing Research* 28 (6): 726–39.

MAXIMIZING PROFITS

CHAPTER

10

Learning Objectives

After reading this chapter, students will be able to:

- **define** measures of profitability,
- **describe** two strategies for increasing profits,
- **explain** why a firm should expand if marginal revenue exceeds marginal cost,
- **use** a model to choose the profit-maximizing level of output, and
- **discuss** differences between for-profit and not-for-profit providers.

Key Concepts

- All healthcare managers need to understand how to maximize profits.
- Most healthcare organizations are inefficient, so cost reductions can increase profits.
- To maximize profits, expand as long as marginal revenue exceeds marginal cost.
- *Marginal cost* is the change in total cost associated with a change in output.
- *Marginal revenue* is the change in total revenue associated with a change in output.
- Managers need to understand their costs and not confuse incremental cost with average cost.
- The agency problem arises because the goals of stakeholders may not coincide.

10.1 Introduction

Substantial numbers of healthcare managers serve firms that seek to maximize profits. For example, for-profit hospitals, most insurance firms, most physician groups, and a broad range of other organizations explicitly seek maximum profits. In addition, recognizing that "with no margin, there is no mission," many not-for-profit healthcare organizations act like profit-maximizing firms.

And even organizations that are not exclusively focused on the bottom line must balance financial and other goals. Bankrupt organizations accomplish nothing. As a result, even healthcare managers with objectives other than maximizing profits need to understand how to maximize profits. A manager who does not understand the opportunity cost (in terms of forgone profits) of a strategic decision cannot lead effectively. All healthcare managers need to understand what it takes to maximize profits. Finally, as markets become more competitive, the differences between for-profit and not-for-profit firms are likely to narrow.

Profits are the difference between total revenue and total cost. To maximize profits, you must identify the strategy that makes this difference the largest. In other words, identify the product price (or quantity) and characteristics that maximize the difference between total revenue and total cost.

10.2 Cutting Costs to Increase Profits

An obvious way to increase profits is to cut costs. Most healthcare organizations are inefficient, meaning they could produce the same output at less cost or they could produce higher quality output for the same cost. The inference that healthcare organizations are inefficient is based on two types of evidence. First, studies by quality management and reengineering teams have identified that costs can be reduced by increasing the quality of care. For example, a project at New York University Medical Center that reengineered its cardiovascular service more than tripled the number of patients who were discharged in less than seven days and improved the quality of care (as evidenced by a lower readmission rate). The second type of evidence results from statistical studies. For example, a sophisticated study of hospital efficiency concluded that inefficiency represented more than 13 percent of costs (Zuckerman, Hadley, and Iezzoni 1994).

As Table 10.1 illustrates, the payoff from cost reductions can be substantial. The organization in the table earns $40,000 on revenue of $2.4 million. This operating margin (profits/revenue) of 1.7 percent suggests that the organization is not profitable. Reducing costs by only 2 percent changes this picture entirely. As long as the cost cuts represent more efficient operations, all of the cost reductions will increase profits, in this case by 118 percent.

10.2.1 Cost Reduction Through Improved Clinical Management
Cost reductions often require improvements in clinical management because differences in costs are primarily driven by differences in resource use, not differences in the cost per unit of resource. (An organization cannot

Case 10.1	**Perfecting Patient Care**

"I recommend we take the Lean production approach and apply process redesign to our nursing home," said Jordan. "This approach will help us reduce costs, improve employee satisfaction, and attract more residents."

"Thanks, Jordan," said Reilly, the system vice president for finance. "I appreciate your enthusiasm, but my experience has been that cost cutting always involves reducing the quality of care or increasing the pressure on employees. Our strategic vision is not consistent with either of those directions."

"Reilly, I'm going to have to disagree," interjected Lee. "My reading of the management literature on the Toyota Production System in healthcare confirms that Jordan is onto something. Waste pervades this place. We are doing things that residents don't want, and we are doing them inefficiently and unsafely. Eliminating wasted time and wasted materials will make life better for everyone. By teaching our managers how to help workers create safe, efficient work processes, we can transform this facility from a very good nursing home to a superb nursing home that makes lots of money. There is plenty of evidence that nursing homes are not efficient (Laine et al. 2005; Vitaliano and Toren 1994), and the approach that Jordan is recommending has worked in hospitals (Thompson, Wolf, and Spear 2003)."

Discussion questions:

- Why is inefficiency common in healthcare? Doesn't competition force organizations to be efficient?
- What evidence do we have that process redesign can improve efficiency? Isn't process redesign just another name for making employees work harder? Is there evidence that employees will accept the redesign?
- There is plenty of evidence that quality of care problems harm patients, but won't improving quality cost more? How could better quality not cost more?

	Status Quo	*2% Cost Reduction*
Quantity	24,000	24,000
Revenue	$2,400,000	$2,400,000
Cost	$2,360,000	$2,312,800
Profit	$40,000	$87,200

TABLE 10.1
The Effects of Cost Reductions on Profits

maximize profits if it overpays for the resources it uses.) In turn, differences in resource use are driven by differences in how clinical plans are designed and executed. Improvements in clinical management require physician cooperation and, more typically, physician involvement. Even though many healthcare professionals make clinical decisions, physicians in most settings have a primary role in decision making.

Having recognized the importance of physicians in increasing efficiency, managers need to ask whether the interests of the organization and its physicians are aligned. In other words, will changes that benefit the organization also benefit its physicians? If not, physicians cannot be expected to be enthusiastic participants in these activities, especially if the advantages for patients are not clear.

Managers are responsible for ensuring that the interests of individual physicians are aligned with the organization or for changing the environment. For example, physicians usually benefit from changes in clinical processes that improve the quality of care or make care more attractive to patients. If the change proposal is presented in this fashion, physicians may understand how they will benefit from the improvements. In other cases, however, physicians cannot be expected to participate in quality improvement activities without compensation. For independent physicians, explicit payments for participation may be required. The same may be true for employee physicians, or participation may be a part of their contractual obligations. In both cases, managers must be aware of the high opportunity cost of time spent away from clinical practice.

Where feasible, physician compensation can incorporate bonuses based on how well they meet or exceed clinical expectations. This system helps align the incentives of the organization and its physicians, and it is a continuing reminder to improve clinical management.

10.2.2 Reengineering

Reengineering and quality improvement initiatives can increase profits, but that does not mean they will or that they will do so easily. Nothing guarantees that costs will fall, and nothing guarantees that revenues will not fall faster than costs. Especially in hospitals, improvement initiatives often coincide with downsizing efforts, making the staff wary (and sometimes causing the organization to lose the employees it most wants to keep).

Skilled leadership does not guarantee success but is essential to improvement initiatives. A recent study of hospitals that embarked on reengineering projects found that, two years after implementation, the typical hospital experienced modest improvements in profitability, a substantial number experienced significant improvements, and a similar number experienced significant deterioration (Serb 1998). Reengineering and quality

---

Sidebar 10.1 Profiting from Clinical Improvement

Hospitals usually are paid more when patients experience complications (although Medicare has proposed to end reimbursement for some clinical shortcomings). Because their incremental revenues are highly visible and incremental costs are not, hospitals may think that clinical shortcomings are not eroding margins. A recent analysis of surgical complications (Dimick et al. 2006) should help dispel that notion. Colon resection without complications resulted in costs of $15,464 and a profit margin of 31 percent. When complications occurred, costs more than doubled and the profit turned into a 4 percent loss. Abdominal aortic aneurism repair without complications entailed costs of $22,822 and a profit margin of 26 percent. With complications, costs nearly tripled and the margin fell to 11 percent. Ventral incisional hernia repair without complications cost $6,321 and produced a profit margin of 19 percent. If complications occurred, costs nearly doubled and the margin fell to 6 percent.

Poor quality reduces hospital profits, even though it substantially increases payments by insurers. Given the substantial incentives for insurers and hospitals to reduce complications, good managers should be collaborating to improve outcomes.

---

management initiatives demand the time and attention of everyone in the organization, meaning that other things are left undone or are done less well. If not done skillfully, reengineering and quality management initiatives can make things worse.

10.3 Maximizing Profits

Organizations can also increase profits by expanding or contracting output. The basic rules of profit maximization are to expand as long as marginal revenue exceeds marginal cost, to shrink as long as marginal cost exceeds marginal revenue, and to shut down if the return on investment is not adequate. If increasing output increases revenue more than costs, profits rise. If reducing output reduces costs more than it reduces revenue, profits rise.

What are marginal cost and marginal revenue (or incremental cost and incremental revenue)? *Marginal cost* is the change in total cost associated with a change in output. *Marginal revenue* is the change in total revenue associated with a change in output. The challenges lie in forecasting revenues and estimating costs.

TABLE 10.2

Marginal Cost, Marginal Revenue, and Profits

Quantity	Revenue	Cost	Profit	Marginal Revenue	Marginal Cost
100	$2,000	$1,500	$500		
120	$2,400	$1,600	$800	$20	$5
140	$2,660	$1,840	$820	$13	$12
160	$2,880	$2,120	$760	$11	$14

As shown in Table 10.2, increasing output from 100 to 120 increases profits because the marginal revenue is greater than the marginal cost. Revenue increases from $2,000 to $2,400 as sales increase from 100 to 120 units, so marginal revenue equals $20 ($400 ÷ 20). Costs increase from $1,500 to $1,600, so marginal cost equals $5 ($100 ÷ 20). The same is true for the expansion from 120 to 140. Marginal revenue fell because the firm had to cut prices to increase sales, and marginal cost rose because the firm is approaching capacity. Even though marginal revenue is nearly equal to marginal cost, profits still rose. Expanding from 140 to 160 reduced profits. Further price cuts pushed marginal revenue below marginal cost.

10.3.1 Incremental and Average Costs

Managers need to understand what their costs are and must not confuse incremental costs with average costs. Average costs may be higher or lower than incremental costs. As long as the organization is operating well below capacity, average costs usually will exceed incremental costs because of fixed costs. As the firm approaches capacity, however, incremental costs can rise quickly. If the firm needs to add personnel, acquire new equipment, or lease new offices to serve additional customers, incremental cost may well exceed average costs.

The following example illustrates why managers need to understand marginal costs and compare them to marginal revenues. A clinic is operating near capacity when it is approached by a small preferred provider organization (PPO). The PPO wants to bring 100 additional patient visits to the clinic and pay $50 per visit. The manager accepts the deal, even though $50 is less than the clinic's average cost or average revenue. Shortly thereafter, another PPO approaches the clinic. It too wants to bring 100 additional patient visits to the clinic and pay $50 per visit. The manager turns down the offer. When criticized for this apparent inconsistency, the manager defends herself, explaining that the clinic had excess capacity when it was contacted by the first PPO. The marginal cost for those additional visits was only $10 (see Table 10.3). Signing the first contract increased profits by $4,000,

TABLE 10.3

Marginal Cost and Profits

	Status Quo	Adding the First PPO	Adding the Second PPO
Quantity	24,000	24,100	24,200
Revenue	$2,400,000	$2,405,000	$2,410,000
Average Revenue	$100.00	$99.79	$99.59
Marginal Revenue		$50.00	$50.00
Cost	$2,040,000	$2,041,000	$2,092,000
Average Cost	$85.00	$84.69	$86.45
Marginal Cost		$10.00	$510.00
Profit	$360,000	$364,000	$318,000

because the marginal revenue was $50 for those visits. When the second PPO contacted the clinic, it no longer had excess capacity and would have had to add staff to handle the additional visits. As a result, marginal costs for the second set of visits would have been $510, and profits would have plummeted.

10.4 Return on Investment

When examining an entire organization rather than a well-defined project, most analysts focus on return on equity rather than return on investment. *Equity* is an organization's total assets minus outside claims on those assets. Equity also can be defined as the initial investments of stakeholders (donors or investors) plus the organization's retained earnings.

What is an adequate return on investment? The answer to this question depends primarily on three factors: what low-risk investments are yielding (such as short-term U.S. Treasury securities), the riskiness of the enterprise, and the objectives of the organization.

All business investments entail some risk. Those risks may be high, as they are for a pharmaceutical company considering allocating research and development funds to a new drug, or they may be low, as they are for a primary care physician purchasing an established practice in a small town. In any case, a profit-seeking investor will be reluctant to commit funds to a project that promises a rate of return similar to the yield of low-risk securities. Consequently, when rates of return on low-risk investments are high, investors will demand high yields on higher-risk investments. The size of this risk premium will usually depend on a project's perceived risk. An investor may be content with the prospect of a 9 percent return on investment from a relatively low-risk enterprise but will not find this yield adequate for a high-risk venture.

Because managers must be responsive to the organization's stakeholders, they must also avoid high-risk investments that do not offer at least a chance of high rates of return. What constitutes a high rate of return depends on the goals of the organization and the nonfinancial attributes of an investment. In some cases, an organization that is genuinely committed to nonprofit objectives will be willing to accept a low return (or even a negative return) on a project that furthers those goals.

10.5 Producing to Stock or to Order

Organizations can produce to stock or to order. One that produces to stock forecasts its demand and cost and produces output to store in inventory. Medical supply manufacturers are an example of this sort of organization. More commonly in the healthcare sector, firms produce to order. They also forecast demand and cost, but they do not produce anything up front. Instead, they set prices designed to maximize profits and wait to see how many customers they attract. Hospitals are an example of this type of organization. This distinction is important because discussions of profit maximization are usually framed in terms of choosing quantities or choosing prices.

Thus far, the content of this chapter has been largely framed in terms of firms that produce to stock; however, its implications apply to healthcare organizations that produce to order. Only by setting prices based on their expectations about demand and cost do they discover whether they have set prices too high or too low. An organization has set prices too high if its marginal revenue is greater than its marginal cost, because that means additional profitable sales at a lower price were missed. An organization has set prices too low if its marginal revenue is less than its marginal cost. Organizations that produce to order must also make the same decisions about rates of return on equity discussed earlier. Is the 5 percent return on investment large enough to justify operating an organ transplant unit? How important is the unit to the organization's educational goals? What are the alternatives?

When organizations contract with insurers or employers, estimates of marginal revenue should be easy to develop. They calculate projected revenue under the new contract, subtract revenue under the old contract, and divide by the change in volume. For sales to the general public, economics gives managers a tool: marginal revenue = $p \times (1 + 1/\varepsilon)$, where p is the product price and ε is the price elasticity of demand. (See Chapter 7 for more information about elasticity.) Most healthcare organizations face price elasticities in the range of –3.00 to –6.00, so marginal revenue can be much less than the price. For example, if a product sells for $1,000 and the price elasticity of demand is –3.00, its marginal revenue will equal $1,000 × (1 – 1/3.00), or $667. In contrast, if the price elasticity of demand is –6.00, its marginal revenue will equal $1,000 × (1 – 1/6.00), or $833. As you can see, as demand becomes more elastic, marginal revenue and price become more alike. Unless the elasticity becomes infinite, though, marginal revenue will be less than price.

10.6 Not-for-Profit Organizations

The strategies of not-for-profit organizations may differ from those of for-profit organizations because of more severe *agency* problems, and goals and costs specific to not-for-profit status. These forces have different effects on profits and obscure the extent of ownership's influence on outcomes.

10.6.1 Agency Problems

All organizations have agency problems. Agency problems are conflicts between the interests of managers (the agents) and the goals of other stakeholders. For example, a higher salary benefits a manager, but it benefits stakeholders only if it enhances performance or keeps the manager from leaving (when a comparable replacement could not be attracted for less). Not-for-profit firms face three added challenges. They cannot turn managers into owners by requiring them to own company stock (which helps to align the interests of managers and other owners). In addition, no one owns the organization, so no one may be policing the behavior of its managers to ensure they are serving stakeholders well. Furthermore, assessing the performance of managers in not-for-profit organizations is a challenge. A not-for-profit organization may earn less than a for-profit competitor for many reasons. Is it earning less because of its focus on other goals, because of management's incompetence, or because the firm's managers are using the firm's resources to live well? Often the cause is difficult to pinpoint.

10.6.2 Differences in Goals

Goals other than profits can influence an organization's behavior, though they need not. Not-for-profit firms gain benefits from the pursuit of goals other than profit. Managers should consider how their decisions affect the benefits derived from these other goals. To best realize its goals, a not-for-profit organization should strive to make marginal revenue + marginal benefit equal to marginal cost. *Marginal benefit* is the net marginal benefit to the firm from expanding a line of business. Three cases are possible:

1. If the marginal benefit > 0, the not-for-profit will produce more than a for-profit.
2. If the marginal benefit = 0, the not-for-profit will produce as much as a for-profit.
3. If the marginal benefit < 0, the not-for-profit will produce less than a for-profit.

A further complication is that the marginal benefit may depend on other income. A struggling not-for-profit may act like a for-profit, but a highly profitable not-for-profit may not.

10.6.3 Differences in Costs

Not-for-profit organizations' costs also may differ. First, the not-for-profit may not have to pay taxes (especially property taxes), which tends to make the not-for-profit's average costs lower. On the other hand, the not-for-profit firm's greater agency problems may result in less efficiency and higher average and marginal costs.

The fundamental problem is that we cannot predict how not-for-profit organizations will differ from for-profit firms. This lack of forecast is frustrating for analysts and raises a question for policymakers: If we do not know how not-for-profit organizations benefit the community, why are they given tax breaks?

10.7 Conclusion

Even managers of not-for-profit organizations need to know how to maximize profits. They must identify appropriate product lines, price and promote those product lines to realize an adequate return on investment, and produce those product lines efficiently. Most healthcare organizations are less profitable than they could be because they are less efficient than they could be. Leadership must be effective for efficiency to increase. Cost reductions and quality improvements are easier to talk about than realize, especially where clinical plans (i.e., physician practices) must change to improve efficiency.

Decisions to expand or contract should be based on incremental costs and revenues. Few healthcare managers know what their costs are, so they often have difficulty forecasting revenues and estimating costs to be able to make these decisions.

Not-for-profit organizations may or may not resemble for-profit organizations. In some cases, their goals and performance are similar. Managers need to understand why the goals of not-for-profit organizations are worthy of tax preferences and be able to make that case to donors and regulators.

| Case 10.2 | Tax Exemption for Nonprofit Hospitals |

"Tax exemption for nonprofit hospitals is a historical relic," said Tyler at a hospital board meeting. "When income tax started in 1894, there was no Medicare, no Medicaid, and no insurance. People with money got care at home. The role of hospitals was to care for the poor. These days, hospitals are profitable businesses that serve paying customers. Even lobbyists for the industry concede that that exemption from federal, state, and local taxes almost certainly costs more than the care nonprofit hospitals provide for free to the poor. For-profits, which pay income and property taxes, provide about as much uncompensated care as nonprofits. Plus, a lot of free care is mandatory. Federal and state laws require all hospitals to provide emergency care without regard for ability to pay.

"Look, well-run 'nonprofits' make plenty of money, and their managers get paid very well. I have no problem with that, but they shouldn't get a tax break, too." With that, Tyler sat down.

Kim then approached the microphone, saying, "I know that we provide charity care. But Suburban Clinic, which is for-profit and pays local property taxes, does too. And it provides only a little less than we do. A first guess at our property value would be $60 million. The local taxes on that would be about $1.8 million. Even using the inflated estimates that we float, which are based on list prices, there's no way that its community benefit approaches that amount of money. Have you seen the roads in this town? We could really use the tax revenue. And I wouldn't mind a tax cut. My taxes help pay for our nonpayment of taxes. You know, we bought three for-profit physician practices, and I see no difference in the way they are run. I think this is just a scam to avoid paying taxes."

After Kim sat down, Lee, the hospital's CEO, took the floor. "We provide a broad array of benefits to this community. We provide charity care, our prices are lower than our competitors, we operate a nursing school, we operate asthma and heart failure programs that consistently lose money, and we operate a number of community outreach programs. I think this community is well served by its recognition of our charitable mission. Yes, we are profitable, but we need to stay in business. I look forward to working with the board of assessors to clear up any questions about the merits of our nonprofit status. I am confident that they are based on a misunderstanding of the situation."

Several more speakers came to the microphone, but none brought a lot of new information. Next, the board of assessors had to make a decision about the status of the hospital.

(continued)

Case 10.2 continued

Discussion questions:

- What evidence is there about the level of community benefit provided by nonprofit and for-profit hospitals? Why does using list prices tend to inflate estimates of community benefit? Are there other important differences between nonprofit and for-profit hospitals?
- Would the city be better off if it taxed the hospital and paid for charity care? More broadly, is tax exemption a good way to encourage private organizations to serve the public interest?
- What should the board of assessors do? What are its options?

Homework

10.1 A clinic has $1 million in revenues and $950,000 in costs. What is its operating margin?

10.2 The owners of the clinic invested $400,000. What is the return on investment? Is it adequate?

10.3 A laboratory has $4.2 million in revenues and $3.85 million in costs. What is its operating margin?

10.4 The owners of the laboratory invested $6 million. What is the return on investment?

10.5 Go to www.federalreserve.gov/. What is the current annual yield for one-year Treasury securities?

10.6 Go to http://finance.yahoo.com/q/ks?s=cyh and look up the operating margin, return on assets, and return on equity for Community Health Systems (symbol = CYH). How does it compare to Aetna (AET), Amgen (AMGN), Laboratory Corporation of America (LH), and Tenet Healthcare Corporation (THC)?

10.7 A not-for-profit hospital realizes a 3% return on its $200,000 investment in its home health unit. Its current revenue after discounts and allowances is $382,000. Administrative costs are $119,000; clinical personnel costs are $210,000; and supply costs are $47,000. Providing home health care is not a core goal of the hospital, and it will sell the home health unit if it cannot realize a return of at least 12 percent. A process improvement team has recommended significant changes to the home health unit's billing processes. The team has concluded that these changes could reduce costs by $20,000 and increase revenues by $5,000. Analyze the data that follows and assess whether they would make the home health unit profitable enough to keep.

	Old	New
Revenue	$382,000	$387,000
Cost	$376,000	$356,000
Profit	$6,000	$31,000
ROI	3%	16%

10.8   Below are cost and revenue data for an outpatient surgery clinic. Calculate its marginal cost, marginal revenue, and profits at each level of output. Which price maximizes its profits?

Surgeries	250	300	350	400	450
Price	$2,000	$1,920	$1,800	$1,675	$1,550
Revenue	$500,000	$576,000	$630,000	$670,000	$697,500
Cost	$516,000	$538,500	$563,500	$591,000	$621,000

10.9   The price–quantity relationship has been estimated for the new prostate cancer blood test: $Q = 4,000 - (20 \times P)$. Use a spreadsheet to calculate the quantity demanded and total spending for prices ranging from $200 to $0, using $50 increments. For each $50 drop in price, calculate the change in revenue, the change in volume, and the additional revenue per unit. Call the additional revenue per unit marginal revenue.

10.10 Below are output and cost data. Calculate the average total cost (ATC), average fixed cost (AFC), average variable cost (AVC), and marginal cost (MC) schedules. If the market price were $500, should the firm shut down in the short run? In the long run?

Quantity	0	5	10	15	20	25	30	35
Total Cost	$20,000	$20,500	$20,975	$21,425	$21,850	$22,300	$22,775	$23,275

10.11 A clinic's average and marginal cost per case is $400. It charges $600 per case and serves 1,000 customers. Its marketing team predicts that it will expand its sales to 1,250 customers if it cuts its price to $550. How do profits change if it cuts prices? What is the firm's marginal revenue? Why is marginal revenue not equal to $550?

10.12 A clinic's average and marginal cost per case is $400. It charges $600 per case and serves 1,000 customers. Its marketing team predicts that it will expand its sales to 1,250 if it signs a contract for a price of $550 with a local health maintenance organization. How do profits change if it signs the contract? What is the firm's marginal revenue? Why is its marginal revenue different from the marginal revenue in the previous problem?

10.13 Why would a for-profit organization that incurs losses choose to operate?

10.14 Why would a for-profit organization that is earning profits choose to exit a line of business?

Chapter Glossary

Marginal or incremental cost. The cost of producing an additional unit of output

Marginal revenue. The revenue from selling an additional unit of output

Production to order. Setting prices and then filling customers' orders

Production to stock. Producing output and then adjusting prices to sell what has been produced

Profits. Total revenue minus total cost

Return on assets. Profits divided by assets

Return on equity. Profits divided by shareholder equity

References

Dimick, J. B., W. B. Weeks, R. J. Karia, S. Das, and D. A. Campbell. 2006. "Who Pays for Poor Surgical Quality? Building a Business Case for Quality Improvement." *Journal of the American College of Surgeons* 202 (6): 933–37.

Laine, J., M. Linna, A. Noro, and U. Häkkinen. 2005. "The Cost Efficiency and Clinical Quality of Institutional Long-Term Care for the Elderly." *Health Care Management Science* 8 (2): 149–56.

Serb, C. 1998. "Is Remaking the Hospital Making Money?" *Hospitals & Health Networks* 72 (14): 32–33.

Thompson, D. N., G. A. Wolf, and S. J. Spear. 2003. "Driving Improvement in Patient Care: Lessons from Toyota." *Journal of Nursing Administration* 33 (11): 585–95.

Vitaliano, D. F., and M. Toren. 1994. "Cost and Efficiency in Nursing Homes: A Stochastic Frontier Approach." *Journal of Health Economics* 13 (3): 281–300.

Zuckerman, S., J. Hadley, and L. Iezzoni. 1994. "Measuring Hospital Efficiency with Frontier Cost Functions." *Journal of Health Economics* 13 (3): 255–80.

PRICING

After reading this chapter, students will be able to:

- **apply** the standard marginal cost pricing model,
- **explain** why price discrimination can increase profits,
- **explain** the link between pricing and profits, and
- **discuss** the importance of price setting.

- Pricing is important.
- *Marginal cost pricing* maximizes profits in most cases.
- Marginal cost pricing uses estimates of the price elasticity of demand and incremental costs to set the profit-maximizing price.
- The consequences of setting prices incorrectly can be substantial.
- *Price discrimination* is common in healthcare and other industries.
- Price discrimination can substantially increase profits.
- Contracting demands the same information as pricing.

11.1 Introduction

Pricing is important. Prices set too low or too high will drag down profits. The trick is to set prices so your organization captures profitable business and discourages unprofitable business. To maximize profits, marginal revenue should just equal marginal cost (assuming the product line is profitable). To maximize other objectives, organizations should start with profit-maximizing prices.

Pricing is a continuing challenge for healthcare organizations for three reasons. First, many managers do not have a clear pricing strategy. They lack the necessary data to make good decisions and may be mispricing their products or selling the wrong product lines. Second, many healthcare organizations have jumped directly from the hothouse of cost-plus or reimbursement-plus pricing to the real world of competitive bidding and contract negotiation. They lack skills and experience in setting prices and negotiating contracts. Third, the pricing strategy that is best for the organization may not be the pricing strategy various departments or clinics prefer. Managers of these units may have incentives to price products too high or too low. In the absence of a clear strategy and good data, how prices will actually be set will be up for grabs.

11.2 The Economic Model of Pricing

The economic model of pricing, *marginal cost pricing,* clearly identifies a pricing strategy that will maximize profits. This strategy also identifies the information needed to set prices.

The economic model of pricing is quite simple. First, find out what your incremental costs are. (Remember, incremental costs are the same as marginal costs.) Second, estimate the price elasticity of demand facing *your organization's product.* (Demand for the products of your organization will usually be much more elastic than the overall demand for the product. See Chapter 7 for more information about elasticity.) Third, calculate the appropriate markup, which will equal $\varepsilon/(1 + \varepsilon)$. (Here, ε represents the price elasticity of demand for your organization's product.) Multiplying this markup times your organization's incremental cost gives you the profit-maximizing price. The profit-maximizing price will equal $[\varepsilon/(1 + \varepsilon)] \times MC$, where MC represents the incremental cost. So, if the price elasticity of demand is -2.5 and the incremental cost is $3.00, the profit-maximizing price would be $[-2.5/(1 - 2.5)] \times 3.00$, or $5.00.

By now you may have noted that the pricing rule is just a restatement of the profit maximization rule from Chapter 10, which states that marginal revenue equals marginal cost, $MR = MC$. The formula for marginal revenue is $\text{Price} \times (1 + \varepsilon)/\varepsilon$, so $MC = \text{Price} \times (1 + \varepsilon)/\varepsilon$. Solve this formula for Price by dividing both sides by $(1 + \varepsilon)/\varepsilon$, and you end up with $\text{Price} = MC/(1 + \varepsilon)/\varepsilon$, which is the same as $[\varepsilon/(1 + \varepsilon)] \times MC$.

Data on incremental costs are important for a wide range of management decisions. Pricing is one more reason to estimate incremental costs. Estimating the right price elasticity of demand can be more of a challenge. Three strategies can provide you with this information. One would be to hire a marketing consultant. Depending on how much your organization is willing to spend, the consultant can provide you with a rough or fairly detailed estimate. Another strategy would be to combine information on overall market price elasticities of demand with information on your market share for this product line. (Chapter 7 lists a number of market price elasticities.) Dividing the overall price elasticity of demand by your market share gives an estimate of the price elasticity your organization faces. For example, if the overall price elasticity is –0.3 and your organization commands an eighth of the market, you would estimate that your organization faces a price elasticity of demand of –0.3/0.125, or –2.4. The third strategy would be to experiment. For example, raise a product's price by 5 percent and see how much demand falls. Since the price elasticity of demand equals the percentage change in quantity sold divided by the percentage change in price, this calculation is straightforward.

Table 11.1 illustrates how different profit-maximizing markups can be. An organization facing a price elasticity of demand of –2.5 and an incremental cost of $10.00 should have a markup of $6.67. In contrast, a similar organization facing a price elasticity of demand of –5.5 should set a markup of $2.22. Each of these choices maximizes profits, given the market environment each firm faces. Clearly, organizations that face less elastic demand enjoy larger markups. The payoffs to differentiating your products can be substantial, since these products face less elastic demand.

11.3 Pricing and Profits

What should you do if the rate of return from a line of business is inadequate? The obvious solution is to raise prices. Unfortunately, like many obvious strategies, this one will often be wrong. If a product line yields an inadequate return on investment, four strategies should be explored.

1. Make sure your price is not too high or too low. Return to the maximum pricing formula and see if you calculated incorrectly, or whether your estimate of the price elasticity of demand was inaccurate.

Elasticity	Price
–1.5	$30.00
–2.5	$16.67
–3.5	$14.00
–4.5	$12.86
–5.5	$12.22
–6.5	$11.82
–7.5	$11.54
–8.5	$11.33
–9.5	$11.18

TABLE 11.1

Profit-Maximizing Prices When Incremental Costs Equal $10

2. Reassess your estimate of incremental costs. If it is too high, your prices will also be too high, and vice versa.
3. See how much you can cut your costs. Most healthcare firms should be able to reduce costs quite substantially. To see whether yours can be brought down, take a look at costs and business practices in firms you think are efficient.
4. If all else fails, exit the line of business.

The consequences of setting price incorrectly can be substantial. In Table 11.2 the profit-maximizing price should be $15.00. Setting a price much lower or much higher than $15.00 reduces profits significantly. Note, though, that being a bit too high or a bit too low is not disastrous. Being a little off in your estimates of incremental cost or the price elasticity of demand will usually mean your profits will be little smaller than they could have been.

Pricing is an important component of marketing. How is the marginal cost pricing model outlined above too simple? The main concern is that it does not account for strategy. For example, demand for an innovative product will typically be quite inelastic. The resulting high margins, unfortunately, will attract a host of rivals. Your organization may want to forgo some immediate profits to discourage entry by competitors. Alternatively, aggressive price cutting in mature markets is likely to encourage price cutting by your competitors. In markets with relatively few competitors, not rocking the boat by cutting prices may allow everyone to enjoy stable, high prices and high profits. These factors demand careful study, but even if you do not follow the marginal cost pricing scenario, it should be your starting point.

TABLE 11.2
Profits When Incremental and Average Costs Equal $10 and the Price Elasticity of Demand Equals –3.0

Price	Profits
$5.00	($881,059)
$7.50	($130,527)
$10.00	$0
$12.50	$28,194
$15.00	$32,632
$17.50	$30,824
$20.00	$27,533
$22.50	$24,172
$25.00	$21,145

11.4 Price Discrimination

Price discrimination is common in healthcare, as it is in other industries. *Price discrimination* refers to charging different customers different prices for the same product. Price discrimination makes sense if different customers have different price elasticities of demand and if resale of the product by customers is not possible. Most healthcare providers and their products meet these criteria. They contract with an array of individuals and insurance plans. The price sensitivities of those purchasers differ widely, and services can seldom be resold. So, profit-maximizing healthcare firms will want to explore opportunities for price discrimination (or more politely, different discounts for different customers).

Price discrimination can increase profits. Suppose half your customers (group A) have price elasticities of –3.00 and half (group B) have price elasticities of –6.00. The demand curve for group A is 16,000 – 800 × Price, and the demand curve for group B is 16,000 – 1,045 × Price. (You can verify that the group A elasticity is –3.00 at a price of $15.00 and the group B elasticity is –6.00 at a price of $12.00.) Your average and incremental cost is $10. In setting prices you could use the average price elasticity of demand (–4.50) and charge everyone $12.86. Or you could charge group A $12.00 and charge group B $15.00 (which is what the marginal cost pricing model tells us to do). As Table 11.3 illustrates, not price discriminating leaves a substantial amount on the table.

So, aside from managers (who are eager to learn new ways to improve profits) and consumers (who are eager to learn new ways to get discounts), why should price discrimination matter to anyone? Some observers think the different prices reflect *cost shifting*, not price discrimination. According to the cost shifting hypothesis, price reductions negotiated by PPOs or imposed by Medicaid will raise costs for everybody else. The cost shifting hypothesis is widely believed. For example, in 2006 the *New York Times* reported employers and consumers were paying billions more each year because Medicare and Medicaid payments were not rising fast enough (Freudenheim 2006).

The cost shifting hypothesis might be true, but probably is not. Most of the empirical evidence from the contemporary marketplace is inconsistent with the cost shifting hypothesis (Morrisey 1994). Why does the hypothesis persist? There are three possibilities. First, the cost shifting hypothesis may be a rationalization for widespread discounting. No customer likes getting the smallest discount, so perhaps healthcare firms lead the customer to believe his small discount is due to cost shifting ("We could give you a better price if it weren't for the big discount we're forced to give Medicare!"). This is the most likely scenario. Second, cost shifting might be real, reflecting poor management on the part of profit-seeking

| Case 11.1 | **Price Discrimination in Practice** |

What do American Airlines, GlaxoSmithKline, Staples, Stanford University, AT&T, the Mayo Clinic, and Safeway have in common? They all price discriminate, says Scott Woolley (1998). They charge different customers different amounts for the same product.

Pharmaceutical discounts are the clearest examples of healthcare price discrimination, because the products are identical. Only the prices differ.

A cash customer (e.g., someone without insurance coverage) would pay the highest price, the list price. In pharmaceutical jargon, list price is called average wholesale price or AWP.

Most customers pay much less than AWP. Pharmacy benefit managers negotiate discounts with manufacturers and pharmacies. These discounts are typically about 20 percent (von Oehsen, Ashe, and Duke 2003). Some hospitals and HMOs have their own pharmacies and can negotiate even better deals with manufacturers. These organizations often pay as little as 60 percent of AWP.

The federal government has five discount programs. The largest is the Medicaid rebate program, which requires manufacturers to pay a rebate equal to 15.1 percent of their "best" price. The Medicaid price is usually about 60 percent of AWP after the rebate is subtracted.

Many federally funded clinics and hospitals are eligible for the Medicaid discount. However, these agencies can often negotiate better deals because they can buy wholesale and because they can choose drugs for their formularies. These agencies typically pay 50 percent of AWP.

Tribal and territorial governments can use the prices on the Federal Supply Schedule, which federal agencies use to buy common supplies and services. Most of these prices are also about 50 percent of AWP.

The Department of Defense, the Department of Veterans Affairs, the Public Health Service, and the Coast Guard may get prices that are slightly lower than the Federal Supply Schedule because of a provision called the federal ceiling price. This caps the price using a formula based on private-sector transactions.

Finally, these agencies can try to negotiate prices below the federal ceiling price. The Department of Veterans Affairs (VA), which uses a national formulary, has used its bargaining power to get substantially better prices. In some cases the VA pays 35 percent of AWP.

Discussion questions:
- Why do drug firms give discounts voluntarily?
- Do other healthcare providers routinely give discounts to some customers?
- Why do the uninsured typically pay the highest prices?
- Why would a hospital usually get a better price for a drug than an insurance company?
- Why does the VA get such low prices?
- Suppose a law was enacted that required drug manufacturers to give state Medicaid agencies the same price they negotiated with the Department of Veterans affairs. How would Medicaid and VA prices change?

TABLE 11.3
Profits With
and Without
Price
Discrimination

Group	Without Price Discrimination			With Price Discrimination		
	Price	Quantity	Profit	Price	Quantity	Profit
A	$12.86	5,712	$16,336	$15.00	4,000	$20,000
B	$12.86	2,561	$7,324	$12.00	3,460	$6,920
		8,273	$23,660		7,460	$26,920

organizations. If a firm raised prices for some customers because other customers negotiated a discount, either prices were too low to begin with or the firm was acting imprudently in raising prices. Third, cost shifting might be real, reflecting responses of not-for-profit firms that had set prices lower than a well-managed, for-profit firm would have. However, pressure on the bottom lines of contemporary healthcare organizations— profit and nonprofit—means that, if it existed, cost shifting is probably a thing of the past.

Similar differences are common in other industries with similar characteristics. Have you ever wondered why it makes sense for one passenger to have paid $340 for his flight and another passenger in the same row to have paid $99? Why does it make sense for a matinee to cost half as much as the same movie shown two hours later?

When the incremental cost of production is small, when buyers can be separated into groups that have very different price elasticities of demand, and when resale is not possible, price discrimination is usually profitable. Most healthcare firms fit this profile, so their managers need to know how to price discriminate. This is true for not-for-profit and for-profit firms. With no margin, there is no mission. Price discrimination helps increase margins.

11.5 Multi-Part Pricing

Thus far we have focused on simple pricing models. In fact, there is a wide range of pricing models that may be applicable. One is the multi-part pricing model, in which customers pay a fee to be eligible to use a service and separate additional fees as they use the services. An obvious example would be a managed care plan. The trade-off is that a low entry fee (premium) yields more customers. High copays reduce costs (either increasing profit margins or reducing premiums), but at some point high

Case 11.2   What Should You Charge?

Below is your practice's marketing forecast.

Price	Low-Income Clients	High-Income Clients	Total
$35.75	2,125	14,250	16,375
$35.25	2,375	14,750	17,125
$34.75	2,625	15,250	17,875
$34.25	2,875	15,750	18,625
$33.75	3,125	16,250	19,375
$33.25	3,375	16,750	20,125
$32.75	3,625	17,250	20,875
$32.25	3,875	17,750	21,625
$31.75	4,125	18,250	22,375
$31.25	4,375	18,750	23,125
$30.75	4,625	19,250	23,875
$30.25	4,875	19,750	24,625
$29.75	5,125	20,250	25,375
$29.25	5,375	20,750	26,125
$28.75	5,625	21,250	26,875
$28.25	5,875	21,750	27,625
$27.75	6,125	22,250	28,375
$27.25	6,375	22,750	29,125

Discussion questions:
- By law, you must charge everyone the same price. What do you charge?
- Your costs equal $100,000 plus $20 per visit. What are your revenues, costs, and profits?
- If you could charge low-income and high-income customers different prices, what prices would you charge each group? What would your revenues, costs, and profits be? Would this be ethical? How would you try to identify the two groups? (You cannot do income surveys of your patients.)

copays will drive away customers. The right combination is always a balancing act. A related pricing strategy is tying. Tying links the prices of multiple products. Again, the goal is to balance multiple prices so as to maximize profits.

11.6 Pricing and Managed Care

Are these issues relevant in markets dominated by managed care? Yes. One needs the same information to set a price or to evaluate a contract. It almost

Case 11.3   **Should My Firm Accept This Contract?**

You are the manager of a 20-physician cardiology practice. You are getting ready to advise your board about a proposal for capitated specialty care from a local HMO. Data from your fee-for-service practice show billings per member per month of $100 for visits, $80 for catheterizations, and $115 for lab. The practice owns the labs, and the profits are shared among the partners. Your estimate is that costs (aside from physician income) equal 25 percent of charges.

The proposal from the HMO is for a rate of $275 per member per month. Your immediate reaction is to reject it. Your CFO makes two comments that give you pause. She argues, "Our overhead will drop significantly if we accept this proposal and convert 25 percent of our business to capitation. In addition, we should anticipate that our rates for visits, catheterizations, and tests will drop significantly once we convert."

The flip side of the pricing problem, contracting, is even tougher. Economic models of pricing tell us managers need to know what their incremental costs are, what markup over incremental costs they should expect, and what their rivals will bid. Each of these will be uncertain to some degree, and many healthcare firms have only sketchy cost data. This is especially true for incremental costs, which many firms are not prepared to track. Without good data on incremental costs, managers will be flying blind and may be tempted to base their bids on average costs. This usually costs some profitable business opportunities.

In this case there are only two other cardiology groups in town. You are not sure whether they have been asked to bid or not. Your legal counsel has warned you that direct discussions with your rivals might leave you open to an anti-trust suit.

Discussion questions:

- Why is your initial response to reject the offer?
- Why might overhead go down if you accept the contract?
- Why might utilization rates go down?
- What are the risks of accepting or refusing?
- What should you do next? Should you accept the proposal? Should you make a counteroffer?

never makes sense to accept a contract in which marginal revenue is less than incremental cost because this reduces profit. Such contracts make sense only when these losses are really marketing expenses, and even in these cases the money probably could be better spent elsewhere. Similarly, it almost never makes sense to give a large discount to a buyer who is not sensitive to price. For example, a managed care plan that needs your organization's participation in order to offer a competitive network is not in a good bargaining position and should not get the best discount.

11.7 Conclusion

Pricing is important, but many healthcare firms lack direction. Without a clear model of pricing, managers are unable to realize their firm's goals. They do not know what their incremental costs are or what sort of price elasticity of demand their organization faces. As a result, they do not know what prices to charge. This reduces profits two ways. The organization may have set its prices too high or too low. Alternatively, the organization may be participating in the wrong markets. It may be accepting contracts it should refuse or refusing contracts it should accept.

The economic model of pricing tells managers what they should do. Its implications, moreover, apply to both pricing and contracting, so it remains an important part of every healthcare manager's tool kit. Actually applying this model will not always be easy, but not knowing what to do is harder still.

Price discrimination is everywhere in healthcare, and many organizations rely on it to remain profitable. Profitably price discriminating requires a little more information than setting a single price, so the above comments apply to a greater degree. In addition, many healthcare managers are mesmerized by tales of cost shifting. It is unlikely that cost shifting is responsible for differences in price. If managers genuinely believe it is occurring, however, cost shifting steers them in the wrong direction.

Homework

11.1   The marginal cost pricing model calculates a markup over marginal costs using estimates of the price elasticity of demand. Will any other pricing strategy result in higher profits?

11.2   If cost shifting is just a useful public relations ploy, why does it get so much attention?

11.3   Will raising prices increase the rate of return from a line of business?

11.4   Can you think of a healthcare firm that does not price discriminate (i.e., charge different customers different amounts for the same product)?

11.5   Price discrimination requires the ability to distinguish customers who are the most price sensitive and the ability to prevent arbitrage (resale of your products by customers who buy at low prices). What attributes of healthcare products make these tasks easy to do?

11.6   Your pharmacy provides services to Medicare and PPO patients. You estimate a price elasticity of demand of −2.2 for Medicare patients and −5.3 for PPO patients. Your marginal and average cost for dispensing a prescription is $2. What is the profit-maximizing dispensing fee for Medicare and PPO patients? Why might the price elasticities of demand differ?

11.7 Your dental clinic provides 3,000 exams for private pay patients and 1,000 exams for members of the UMW. Your fixed costs are $50,000 and your incremental cost is $40.

    a. Private pay patients have a price elasticity of demand of −3. What do you charge them?

    b. The UMW has negotiated a fee of $50. Is it profitable to treat members of the UMW?

    c. What would happen to your profits if you stopped treating members of the UMW?

    d. If the UMW negotiated a fee of $45 instead, what would you charge private pay patients?

    e. What does this tell you about cost shifting versus price discrimination?

11.8 You provide therapeutic massage services, focusing on stress reduction services that are not covered by insurance. Your monthly overhead is $2,000. You value your time at $20 per half hour (how long a therapeutic massage takes). Supplies per massage cost $4. You currently charge $75 per massage and have a volume of 100 clients per month. *Therapeutic Massage Today*, your trade journal, says that a 5 percent reduction in prices typically results in a 7.5 percent increase in volume. What would happen to your volume, revenues, and profits if you cut your price to $70? If you raised your price to $80?

11.9 Below are cost and revenue data for Dunes Hospital. Calculate its marginal cost, marginal revenue, and profits at each level of output. What price should it choose?

Case-Mix-Adjusted Price and Volume Data for Dunes Hospital

Admissions	6,552	9,048	9,672	9,984	10,296
Revenue	$52,416,000	$70,574,400	$73,507,200	$73,881,600	$74,131,200
Cost	$42,588,000	$59,264,400	$63,835,200	$66,393,600	$68,983,200
Price	$8,000	$7,800	$7,600	$7,400	$7,200

11.10 Your firm spent $100 million developing a new drug. It has now been approved for sale, and each pill costs $1 to manufacture. Your market research suggests that the price elasticity of demand in the general public is −1.1.

    a. What price do you charge the public?

    b. What would happen to profits if you charged twice as much?

    c. What role does the $100 million in development costs play in your pricing decision?

    d. The Medicaid agency has made a take-it-or-leave-it offer of $2 per pill. Do you accept? Why or why not?

11.11   Why are most healthcare providers able to charge different groups of purchasers different prices for the same products?

11.12   A clinic has incremental costs per case of $10 and overhead costs of $100,000. It faces a price elasticity of demand of –2.
  a.   What is the clinic's profit-maximizing price?
  b.   How would the profit-maximizing price change if overhead costs doubled?
  c.   With excess capacity, would it make sense to serve Medicaid customers for a fee of $16?
  d.   How would the profit-maximizing price change if Medicaid raised its fee to $18?

11.13   You manage a not-for-profit hospital in a competitive market. Suppose you decide to charge less than the profit-maximizing price to your customers.
  a.   What effect would that have on profits?
  b.   What effect would that have on you and your career?

11.14   Assume the price elasticity of demand for physicians' services is –0.2. If your marginal cost per visit is $20, what is your profit-maximizing price if you control 5 percent of the market? What is your profit-maximizing price if you control 15 percent of the market? What lessons do you draw from this?

11.15   A busy urgent care clinic has average costs of $40 and incremental costs of $60.
  a.   How could incremental costs be higher than average costs?
  b.   The clinic charges $80 for a visit. What price elasticity of demand does this imply?
  c.   Volume is currently 200 visits per week. What are the clinic's profits?
  d.   An HMO guarantees at least 10 patients per week. It proposes a fee of $55. Should you accept the contract?
  e.   What happens to profits if you accept?

Chapter Glossary

Cost shifting. The hypothesis that price differences are due to efforts by providers to make up for losses in some lines of business by charging higher prices in other lines of business

Marginal cost pricing. Using information about marginal costs and the price elasticity of demand to set profit-maximizing prices

Price discrimination. Selling similar products to different individuals at different prices

References

Freudenheim, M. 2006. "Low Payments by U.S. Raise Medical Bills Billions a Year." [Online article; retrieved 5/15/08.] www.nytimes.com/2006/06/01/business/01health.html.

Morrisey, M. 1994. *Cost Shifting in Health Care: Separating Evidence from Rhetoric.* Washington, DC: AEI Press.

von Oehsen, W. H., M. Ashe, and K. Duke. 2003. "Executive Summary: Pharmaceutical Discounts Under Federal Law: State Program Opportunities." *American Journal of Health System Pharmacy* 60 (15): 551–53.

Woolley, S. 1998. "I Got It Cheaper Than You." *Forbes* 162 (10): 82–84.

12

ASYMMETRIC INFORMATION AND INCENTIVES

Learning Objectives

After reading this chapter, students will be able to:

- **define** asymmetric information and opportunism,
- **describe** two strategies for aligning incentives,
- **explain** why opportunism is a special management challenge in healthcare, and
- **discuss** challenges in limiting opportunism.

Key Concepts

- *Asymmetric information* is a situation in which one party to a transaction has better information about it than another.
- Asymmetric information allows the better informed party to act opportunistically.
- Asymmetric information is a common problem for managers.
- Aligning incentives helps reduce the problems associated with asymmetric information.
- Concerns about risk, complexity, measurement, strategic responses, and team production limit the extent of incentive-based payments.
- Only a few forms of incentive-based contracts are common in healthcare.

12.1 Asymmetric Information

Asymmetric information confronts healthcare managers in most of their professional roles. Vendors typically know more about the strengths and weaknesses of their products than do purchasers. Employees typically know more about their health problems than do human resource or health plan managers. Subordinates typically know more about the effort they have put into their assignments than do their superiors. Providers typically know more about treatment options than do their patients. In all of these examples, one party, commonly called an *agent*, has better information than another party, commonly called a *principal*. Unless the principal is careful, the agent may take advantage of this information asymmetry—in other words, engage in *opportunism*.

Asymmetric information can result in two types of problems. One is that mutually beneficial transactions may not take place if concern about it is too great. The other is that resources may be wasted because of agents' opportunism or principals' costly precautions. For example, an insurer cannot easily discern whether a treatment is really needed (Arrow 1963). In response, an insurer may not cover services thought likely to be abused, may require substantial consumer payments to restrain demand, or may require prior authorization before providing coverage. As a result, consumers may not use helpful services because they cost too much. Alternatively, the plan, providers, and consumers may experience increased costs due to the requirement for prior authorization. (The insurer must staff the authorization office, the provider must spend time and money getting authorizations, and the consumer is likely to experience delays and repeat visits.) Asymmetric information also affects managers directly. Managers are often poorly informed about the quality, efficiency, and customer satisfaction issues that their subordinates face. But managers are also often poorly informed about whether costs are padded, whether quality problems are avoidable, or whether staffing is adequate. Fearing that subordinates will take advantage of them, managers may require reviews or audits. Both increase costs without directly adding to the output of the organization.

Asymmetric information is a concern when:

1. the interests of the parties diverge in a meaningful way,
2. there is an important reason for the parties to strike a deal, and
3. there are difficulties determining whether the explicit or implicit terms of the deal have been followed.

These circumstances are far from rare. Unfortunately, they are an invitation to act opportunistically.

12.2 Opportunism

Opportunism can take many forms. Crime is one form. For example, deliberately billing a health plan for services that were not actually rendered is a form of opportunism more commonly known as *fraud*. The forms of opportunism that managers deal with are not usually so stark. Cruising the Internet rather than making collection calls, using the supplies budget to refurbish your office, scheduling a physical therapy visit of questionable value to meet volume targets, and referring a patient to a specialist for a problem you could easily handle are also examples of opportunism.

From experience, we know that some individuals are opportunistic some of the time. Some individuals seldom act opportunistically, whereas others often do. As a first step, we try to avoid dealing with those who are the most opportunistic. We then try to set up systems to restrain those who may be tempted. These systems will be imperfect because our ability to anticipate what may happen and how individuals may react is imperfect.

12.2.1 Remedies for Asymmetric Information

Remedies for asymmetric information focus on aligning the interests of the parties or monitoring the behavior of the agent. Changes in incentives are usually part of the preferred strategy because monitoring is usually expensive and nonproductive. For example, healthcare plans are commonly subject to utilization review designed to control use of services. Utilization review rarely changes recommended therapies, however, despite its cost and annoyance. Health plans would love to eliminate utilization review. Without it, a plan would rapidly gain market share because it could increase consumer satisfaction, increase provider satisfaction, and reduce premiums. In addition to being costly, monitoring may be difficult. For example, a product that a vendor honestly recommended may fail or may not meet your needs, or it may work but have features you don't need and cost more than a more suitable product. Monitoring is likely to be only part of the remedy for asymmetric information.

12.2.2 The Special Challenges for Healthcare

The challenges posed by asymmetric information are not unique to healthcare, although their extent poses special problems for healthcare managers. Three features make asymmetric information especially troublesome in the healthcare sector:

1. By paying the bills of healthcare providers, insurance creates a principal–agent relationship not found in most fields.
2. Insurance reduces the patient's incentive to monitor the performance of healthcare providers, as it limits the patient's exposure to financial opportunism.
3. Asymmetric information is intrinsic to most provider–patient relationships. Patients typically seek providers' services because they want information, so the threat of opportunism is always present.

Opportunism is such an obvious risk that institutions appear to have developed behaviors to limit it (Arrow 1963). One of the most obvious is our preference for dealing with those who have proven themselves. For example, primary care physicians tend to refer patients to physicians who have served them and their patients well. For fear of losing this business, specialists who might be tempted to provide unnecessary services will be reluctant to do so. These sorts of ongoing relationships—between buyer and seller, patient and provider, and supervisor and subordinate—tend to deter observable opportunism. Much of the regulation of the healthcare sector also serves to deter opportunism. The problem is that these mechanisms work only when opportunism is detectable. In many cases, it is not.

12.2.3 Signaling

When differences in quality or other attributes of care are hard to observe, agents may use signals to reassure principals. These signals should tell prospective clients about the agent, should be hard to counterfeit, and should be relatively inexpensive. Brand names are classic signals. Including a Pfizer label on a new drug costs little and reassures consumers that the drug meets stringent quality standards because substandard quality would hurt Pfizer's sales. The challenge is to prevent others from counterfeiting the labels. Surprisingly, branding in the healthcare market, especially branding of healthcare services, is not that common. Quality certification is another strategy for dealing with asymmetric information. For example, hospital accreditation by The Joint Commission is a signal of quality that is difficult to counterfeit. Unfortunately, the process is so expensive that many smaller hospitals do not seek accreditation.

Other signals may be useful but are likely to be less credible. For example, high prices and high levels of advertising also serve as quality signals, because low-cost, low-quality providers could not afford to advertise frequently or raise prices (Bagwell and Riordan 1991). In markets with standardized products, poorly informed agents can buy information (e.g., by subscribing to *Consumer Reports*) or copy well-informed agents. The more individualized products are, the less this strategy works, so its value in the healthcare market is unclear. Although we can identify healthcare cases in which signaling reduces the problems associated with asymmetric information, it is far from a comprehensive solution.

12.3 Incentive Design for Providers

Recognition that the insurance system of the United States created multiple incentives for inefficiency triggered the growth of managed care. Providers were faced with strong incentives to deliver care as long as the benefits exceeded their patients' costs, and costly care was often free for insured patients. Neither party had a compelling reason for taking the true cost of care into account. We have already discussed redesign of consumer payments, so let's consider how incentives relate to provider payments.

Case 12.1	**Improving Safety**

"Our first priority is improving safety. Some of our nursing homes have very high workers' compensation costs, which just kills the bottom line. Plus, it really gets in the way of providing high-quality care. If workers are shuttling in and out of the nursing home, they cannot build relationships with residents and they will have trouble working together," said our CEO, looking around the table.

Braver than most of us, Dominique honed in on the complex issues this simple idea raised. "Right now we give administrators bonuses and promotions based on profitability. We have to recognize that unsafe work practices may boost productivity; for example, it may take longer to lift patients the safe way. In addition, managers who are working on promoting safety will not be doing the marketing or process improvement work that could boost their facility's profits. It is absolutely true that poor worker safety hurts the system's profits, but it may not hurt the nursing home's profits. After all, the system, not the individual nursing home, pays the workers' compensation premium."

"We have to be smart about this," Casey interjected. "I recently read an article about a restaurant chain that began paying managers a fixed wage plus a share of the restaurant's profits plus a bonus for reducing workers' compensation claims (Puelz and Snow 1997). Some managers improved safety, but some apparently stopped reporting minor accidents (which could get them and us in real trouble). We have to make sure that we get managers to focus on making nursing homes safer places to work, not on convincing workers not to file claims."

Discussion questions:
- Who is the principal and who is the agent in this scenario?
- How is the agent better informed than the principal?
- How do poorly aligned incentives affect the system and individual administrators?
- What could the system do to convince nursing home administrators to improve safety?
- Are financial incentives a part of the action plan? Why or why not?
- How could nursing home administrators signal to the company that they are improving safety?

Incentives are implicit in the four most common methods of paying providers: fee-for-service payments, salaries, capitation, and case rates. Each of these methods has some advantages and disadvantages.

Figure 12.1 contrasts the incentives created by different payment systems. Note that fee-for-service and salary compensation systems incorporate opposite incentives. The incentive structures of capitation and case rate

	Fee-for-Service	Case Rates	Capitation	Salary or Budget
Number of clients	+	+	+	–
Services per client	+	–	–	–
Client acuity*	+	–	–	–
Unbillable services†	–	+	+	+

NOTE: A "+" indicates that the compensation scheme rewards producing more of an output or using more of an input. A "–" indicates that the compensation scheme rewards producing less of an output or using less of an input.

*In this context, client acuity refers to the amount of services that a client is likely to need. Higher acuity means a client is likely to need more services.

†Unbillable services include both services for which the provider cannot bill because of the provisions of the insurance plan and services provided by others.

systems are similar and fall between these opposite cases. Fee-for-service, case rate, and capitation payment systems immediately reward providers who have large numbers of clients. Having more clients means higher revenues in all of these systems. In contrast, unless there are other incentive systems in place (such as review by superiors or the possibility of promotion), salary and budget payment systems do not reward providers according to the number of clients they serve.

The only form of payment that rewards providers who provide a large volume of services per client is fee-for-service payment. In case rate and capitation systems, the disincentive for high volumes of service per client is tempered by the rewards for attracting additional clients. Just as they do not reward for large numbers of clients, salary and budget systems also deter providers from delivering high volumes of service per client.

All of the payment systems except fee-for-service encourage providers to avoid clients with complicated, expensive problems (or at least encourage them to prefer clients with simple, inexpensive problems). Expensive clients, when combined with fixed payments per case or per period, are financially unrewarding for providers. Likewise, all of the payment systems except fee-for-service motivate providers to refer patients to external services (such as church-sponsored organizations or services provided by friends), as long as they are cost-effective from the provider's perspective. From society's perspective, patients should be referred elsewhere as long as the marginal benefit of doing so exceeds the marginal cost. Providers who are paid on the basis of cases, capitation, or salary may refer too often, especially if the provider does not bear the full cost of the services of community organizations or other external services. In contrast, only billable services can be profitable in fee-for-service systems. Fee-for-service creates an incentive not

FIGURE 12.2
An Illustrative
Model of
Incentives

Plan	Base Salary	Marginal Compensation	Volume Payments	Total Income
A	$0	$20	$115,200	$115,200
B	$80,000	$20	$35,200	$115,200
C	$100,000	$20	$35,200	$135,200
D	$57,600	$10	$57,600	$115,200

to use external resources (or at least not to use the organization's resources to improve clients' access to them). Fee-for-service typically rewards providers who refer too infrequently, from society's perspective.

None of these payment systems solves the asymmetric information problem. Providers still usually know more about appropriate treatment options than do patients or insurers. Fee-for-service providers inclined toward opportunism are still able to recommend additional billable services; case rate providers are still able to avoid unprofitable cases; capitated providers are still able to recommend limited treatment plans; and salaried providers are still able to limit how much they do.

This discussion should not be construed as an assertion that only financial incentives matter. Such an assertion would be inconsistent with basic economic theory, which postulates that principals and agents balance alternative objectives. Only some of these goals will be financial. For example, some physicians may offer extensive patient education programs because of their commitment to the health of their patients or because they are an effective marketing tool, even if the fee-for-service payment system does not treat these programs as a billable service. Nonetheless, economics anticipates an aggregate response to financial incentives and predicts that physicians will offer more of such services if the fee-for-service payment system offers compensation for them or if they are profitable under case rate or capitation arrangements.

Suppose that a physician schedules four patients per hour for 30 hours per week and works 48 weeks per year (see Figure 12.2). Under plan A, he earns $20 per patient and has a total income of $115,200. (This example bases compensation on visits to simplify our discussion, not to define an attractive fee-for-service compensation plan. More sensible fee-for-service systems base compensation on billings, relative value units, etc.) Plan B provides a base salary of $80,000 plus $20 per patient for visits in excess of 4,000. At the margin, plans A and B have the same incentives, even though plan B combines salary- and volume-based payments. Each plan pays $20 per patient and provides the same total income. This example illustrates that blended compensation systems can give agents similar incentives with less risk than pure compensation systems.

The incentives of plan C are subtly different from the incentives of plans A and B. Plan C offers a $100,000 base salary plus $20 per patient for visits in excess of 4,000. Although plan C pays $20 per visit at the margin like plans A and B, the physician's income will be higher under plan C than it would be if he saw the same number of patients under plan A or B. Consequently, he may feel less need to add an additional patient at the end of the day or double book to squeeze in an acutely ill patient. In this case, *income effects* are the effects incentive systems have on physicians' decisions about the number of patients they will treat (Rizzo and Blumenthal 1994).

Plan D offers a base salary of $57,600 plus $10 for each patient visit. Even though the physician's income will be the same if he sees 5,760 patients per year under plans A, B, and D, he may choose to see fewer patients under plan D because the marginal reward is smaller.

12.3.1 Insurance and Incentives

How much have compensation systems changed in recent years, given the importance of how providers are paid? Less than you might suspect. For example, even in areas in which managed care is pervasive, most physicians continue to be paid on the basis of their productivity (typically measured by billings, visits, or net revenue), just as they were before the advent of managed care (Robinson et al. 2004). In addition, even though hospital outpatient services represent one of the fastest growing components of medical spending, many health plans continue to pay hospital outpatient departments on the basis of discounted charges (Leary and Farley 2005). This is a surprise because charges seldom reflect costs very accurately (Ginsberg and Grossman 2005). As a result, charge-based payments can make some services very profitable and some services very unprofitable, thereby creating powerful incentives to expand production of some services and curtail production of others.

A striking feature of most insurance plans is payment based on the source of the patient's treatment. Reflecting their historical development, most payment systems are designed to compensate providers. Few are designed to encourage provision of efficient, patient-centered care. Some traditional HMOs might profit by enhancing and integrating care, but most Americans are covered by insurance products that pay individual providers on a fee-for-service basis (Davis and Guterman 2007). For this reason, Medicare's Physician Group Practice demonstration, launched in 2005, was an innovation (Trisolini et al. 2008). This project was designed to reward ten large practices for improving the quality and efficiency of care delivered to Medicare fee-for-service beneficiaries. The demonstration sought to encourage coordination of care, more efficient delivery of services, improved processes, and better outcomes.

12.4 Limits on Incentive-Based Payments

A number of factors limit how complete incentive-based payments can be. Concerns about risk, complexity, and team production make agents reluctant to enter into incentive-based compensation arrangements. Likewise, concerns about opportunism make principals reluctant, as a high-powered incentive system may leave them worse off if agents respond in unanticipated ways.

12.4.1 Risk

Capitation, utilization withholds, and case rate systems are often referred to as *risk-sharing systems*. This term is somewhat misleading. The goal of these systems is incentive alignment; risk sharing is a side effect. For example, capitation gives physicians incentives to use resources wisely, so capitation succeeds if physicians do not run unnecessary tests or if they avoid hospitalizing patients when there are better community treatment options. Full-risk capitation, in which physicians are responsible for all of their patients' costs, gives physicians incentives to take such steps. Unfortunately, the financial risks associated with full-risk capitation can be substantial. One patient with a rare, expensive illness can bankrupt a solo practice; an unexpected jump in pharmaceutical prices can bankrupt a small provider-owned HMO. These risks are one reason capitation's growth has stalled, and many organizations are avoiding full-risk capitation (Terry 2007).

12.4.2 Complexity

Providers and employees are more likely to respond to simple, comprehensible systems than to complex, confusing systems. Simple systems limit the use of incentives and the problems they create. If you want the payment system to reward physicians for keeping customer satisfaction high, MMR (measles, mumps, and rubella) vaccination rates high, out-of-formulary drug use low, hospitalization rates low, hospital lengths of stay short, after-hours response times prompt, record updates prompt, and asthma follow-up appointments timely, the system is likely to be unwieldy. Moreover, the reward associated with each component of the system is likely to be small.

12.4.3 Opportunism

Managers must anticipate opportunistic responses to incentive systems. An agent with better information can harm the principal. In many cases, whether an agent has lived up to contract requirements is difficult to ascertain. In other cases, the agent may act in ways the principal did not anticipate. Some responses will necessitate system redesign; some will have to be tolerated to prevent the system from becoming excessively complex. For example, one response to the price reductions introduced by PPOs was to

Sidebar 12.1 How Much Do Physician Incentives Affect the Use of Expensive Services?

According to a classic study of alternative managed care plans (Josephson and Karcz 1997), incentives have a considerable effect on physicians' use of expensive services. One of the most interesting features of this study is its delineation of how incentives differed for two cohorts of HMO physicians. One cohort of primary care physicians were partners in a capitated, multispecialty group practice that served 22,136 beneficiaries of a large New England HMO. Aside from stop-loss insurance, the physician owners of the practice were at full risk for these beneficiaries' use of services. Unspent capitation funds were distributed to the physicians at the end of the year, so the incentive to keep costs down was significant.

The other cohort of physicians included solo practice physicians who were members of three independent practice association (IPA) HMOs. These physicians were paid on a fee-for-service basis with 10–20 percent withheld. At the end of the year, the withholdings were split equally among the physicians, the hospital, and the HMO. The only risk that these IPA physicians faced was that higher than expected volumes of service per patient would reduce their shares of the withholdings. They also had limited motivation to keep costs down. Fee-for-service payments provided significant incentives to keep volumes (hence costs) up, and the split of the withholding pool weakened their incentives to limit the use of costly services.

The patients of the capitated physicians used fewer emergency department (ED) services. They averaged only 70 visits per thousand members per year. In contrast, the

unbundle services. Physicians and other providers began to bill separately for services once included in the standard office visit. While insurers attempted to limit unbundling in a variety of ways, the fundamental problem remained that the incentives of physicians and insurers were misaligned (Goldfield et al. 2008). Physicians' profits would be higher when they billed for more services, but insurers' profits would be higher when physicians billed for fewer services.

12.4.4 Team Production

Team production also limits the use of incentives. Production of healthcare products usually involves a number of people, and the shortcomings of one person can undermine the efforts of the entire team. For example, rudeness by one disaffected team member can negate the efforts of others to provide exemplary customer service. This interdependency can also weaken the effects of individual incentives. Workers who try hard to do a good job or physicians who are conscientious about reducing length of stay are likely to feel that their efforts are not appreciated if the shortcomings of others deny

patients of the IPA physicians averaged more than five times as many ED visits per year. One reason for this differential was that physicians in the capitated practice operated an after-hours urgent care center to accommodate more than 4,000 patient visits. In addition, the physicians in the capitated practice made a concerted effort to serve walk-in patients during office hours to ensure they were not diverted to the emergency department. In contrast, the IPA physicians, who bore little of the high cost of emergency department care, often referred patients to the emergency department for treatment of unexpected minor illnesses.

Patient incentives, which the study did not consider, may have accounted for some of the difference between the groups. The IPA HMOs may have incorporated weaker incentives for patients to avoid using the emergency department. Although likely to have an impact, differences in patients' incentives do not explain why the prepaid group practice provided comprehensive urgent care services and the IPA practices did not; the physicians decided to provide these services. Capitation aligned the incentives of the physicians and the health plan, as both of them benefited by reducing the use of high-cost emergency department services.

In this case, saving money probably improves the quality of care. In addition to being expensive, care in the emergency department tends to be poorly integrated with other outpatient care. Emergency department physicians may lack timely access to patients' records, and communication with patients' primary care physicians tends to be problematic.

them bonuses. Building and maintaining effective teams are important tasks for managers. Unless carefully structured, financial incentives tend to reward individualistic behavior, which usually weakens teams. Equally problematic, team financial incentives (i.e., every member of the team receives a bonus when the team reaches its goals) often fail to motivate.

12.5 Incentive Design for Managers

Incentives for managers can be financial or nonfinancial. If both types are used, the two incentive systems should operate in tandem. Otherwise, they may worsen the problems created by asymmetric information (Baker, Jensen, and Murphy 1988).

Incentive pay for managers is a partial response to the asymmetric information problem. It usually takes the form of bonus payments, profit sharing, or stock options. In most cases, it is a modest part of total compensation and is only loosely tied to managers' performance.

Sidebar 12.2 Designing a Capitation System

Managed care plans often combine payment methods. Simple strategies, such as capitation without risk adjustment or fee-for-service payments based on discounted charges, create risks that providers are reluctant to assume and incentives that insurers are reluctant to offer. For example, the high cost of treating several patients with AIDS might make a provider reluctant to accept capitation for populations with significant numbers of AIDS patients.

An overview of the Maryland Medicaid risk-adjusted capitation system shows how complicated managed care plans can become (Weiner et al. 1998). The system assigns every beneficiary for whom it has claims information to one of 20 capitation categories. There are 17 diagnosis-based capitation categories with payments ranging from about $45 per month to roughly $1,100 per month. The program assigns new enrollees (for whom it does not have diagnostic data) to capitation groups according to location, age, and sex. The program has separate delivery case and capitation rates for children under age 1. In addition, the program pays a special capitation rate for beneficiaries with AIDS. (The program pays for protease inhibiting drugs and viral load testing on a fee-for-service basis.)

Despite the extensive amount of risk adjustment built into the Maryland program, the program incorporates three mechanisms for limiting the risks borne by healthcare organizations. First, the program has a hospital stop-loss provision. Healthcare organizations are responsible for only 10 percent of annual hospital costs in excess of $61,000 per beneficiary. In addition, the program provides case-managed fee-for-service coverage for beneficiaries with "rare and expensive" conditions (approximately 1 percent of the program population). Spina bifida and cystic fibrosis are examples of these conditions. Third, the program also carves out a behavioral health fee-for-service program. (Persons with psychiatric diagnoses are also assigned high capitation rates for general medical services.) These three provisions address the natural reluctance of healthcare organizations to assume these uncommon but potentially devastating financial risks.

Four concepts underlie incentive pay for managers:

1. Financial incentives can strongly motivate people to perform in ways the organization desires, yet organizations seldom want managers to focus only on duties that will increase their pay. (Fee-for-service compensation presents the same problem.)
2. Managers' goals are often not fully defined. Managers need to respond creatively to problems or, better yet, position the organization to respond to problems that are not yet evident. Performance assessment based on intangibles would be difficult, if not impossible.

3. Most managers' performance is hard to measure. When an individual's productivity becomes hard to measure, compensation based on individual productivity ceases to make sense.

4. What is measurable and what is desired are unlikely to coincide. Compensation based on measurable outputs is likely to increase opportunism, as managers react to what is rewarded rather than to what is sought.

For these reasons, incentive pay for those with significant management roles generally needs to reflect the success of the overall organization. The dilution of incentives that results from using profit sharing or gain sharing is a reasonable price to pay for promoting team-oriented behavior. Gain sharing is like profit sharing but can base bonuses on a broader array of outcomes. Members of a group can earn bonuses for hitting production, customer satisfaction, profit, quality, or cost targets. As individual contributions become less discernable, the more effective group incentives are likely to be. Members of the group will be able to monitor each other more easily, alignment of the group's and organization's incentives will become more important, and the group will more easily alter how it does its work. For example, hospital care is produced by teams, but pay for many physicians depends on their personal billings. To encourage physicians to participate in hospital performance improvement activities, it is often helpful to implement payments to physicians that are based on the performance of the hospital.

Incentive pay is only part of an effective incentive system. Economic theory does not imply that individuals will not respond to opportunities to do challenging work, public celebrations of their accomplishments, or a positive review by a trusted mentor. An effective manager will consider these tools as well. Successful organizations require cooperation in management and production, so a nonfinancial system that rewards cooperation is a sensible option for aligning incentives. Promotions typically combine financial and nonfinancial rewards. Not surprisingly, they are an important part of the reward system in many organizations.

12.6 Conclusion

Incentive restructuring is an imperfect response to the problem of asymmetric information, as are all responses to it. The rewards of incentive systems are usually based on results, not what agents actually do, and agents can respond opportunistically to virtually any incentive system. The challenge is to align the incentives of all the individuals in a system with the interests of

Case 12.2   Using Gain Sharing to Improve Performance

"We could save a lot of money and improve care if we could choose standard cardiology supplies. We could reduce our inventories, negotiate better prices with suppliers, and improve the performance of our surgical teams. Everybody would win," said Cameron.

"Well, not everybody," said Alex, vice president of medical affairs. "Most physicians are more comfortable using a particular type of stent, catheter, or drug. They are familiar with the product, they've used it successfully in the past, and manufacturers are paying some of them to use their products. The article in the *New England Journal of Medicine* by Campbell and colleagues (2007) that we discussed made it pretty clear that drug and device makers use an array of incentives to influence cardiologists. My guess is that it works, or manufacturers would not spend billions on gifts. At a minimum, you need to give a physician a good reason for switching from a familiar drug or device. You also may need to counteract inducements from the manufacturers."

"Our cardiologists are accepting gifts from drug companies and stent manufacturers? That's outrageous," exclaimed Cameron.

"Probably," Alex replied. "It's pretty standard in the field, even though it's a violation of the American Medical Association's code of ethics. It really upsets me, and I'd be willing to work with you to do something about it. But don't kid yourself, if you want to get physicians to adopt a default device or drug, you have to face that the switch will be disruptive for some physicians and will cost them time and money."

At this point, Emerson, the chief legal officer, jumped into the conversation. "Whatever you do, be aware of the concerns of the Health and Human Services Inspector General, who has repeatedly expressed concern about gain-sharing arrangements."

"That's a valid point," replied Alex. "But since 2005 the Inspector General has issued some opinions that permit gain-sharing programs in cardiology. The approved programs all have a clear structure, a plan for sharing gains, a focus on maintaining or improving quality, and a policy of disclosing the gain-sharing program to patients. Ketcham and Furukawa (2008) have studied these programs and concluded that the gain-sharing programs reduced costs and improved quality. My sense is that there's an opportunity here, and we shouldn't shy away from it."

Discussion questions:
- Why would standardization reduce costs? How could it improve quality?
- Could the hospital ban acceptance of samples, gifts, and payments from drug and device makers? Would this be a good strategy? What would the risks be?
- How could the hospital reward physicians for helping standardize cardiology supplies? How would this help align incentives?
- Are any strategies more likely to be effective than others?
- Are any strategies less likely to cause problems with the Inspector General?

its stakeholders. There is no magic formula, as good incentive systems must balance competing objectives. In addition, managers must anticipate that incentives may have multiple effects and that designing incentive systems and keeping them up to date will be expensive.

Homework

12.1 Describe some healthcare situations in which an agent has taken advantage of a principal. Now describe some healthcare transactions that have not taken place because of fears about asymmetric information.

12.2 Identify some ways that nursing homes can signal high quality to consumers. Which of these are most apt to be reliable signals?

12.3 Provide an example of costly monitoring in the healthcare workplace. Can you think of an employment contract that would allow a reduction in monitoring without a reduction in quality?

12.4 What are some strategies for reducing adverse selection in insurance markets? What sorts of problems do these solutions cause?

12.5 One physical therapist is paid $20 per session. Another is paid $400 per week plus $20 per session in excess of 20 sessions per week. A third is paid $400 per week, plus $200 per week for having all paperwork complete and filed within 48 hours, plus $20 per session in excess of 30 sessions per week. How do the therapists' incentives to produce sessions compare? How do their incentives to complete paperwork differ?

12.6 One physician is paid $100 per visit. Another is paid $2,500 per week plus $100 per session in excess of 20 sessions per week. A third is paid $2,000 per week plus $100 per session in excess of 20 sessions per week. The third physician is also paid a weekly bonus of $500 for being in the top quartile in management of common chronic diseases, appropriate antibiotic use, preventive counseling, screening tests, and appropriate prescribing in elderly patients. How do the physicians' incentives compare?

12.7 The Federal Trade Commission requires that firms advertise truthfully. Why does this requirement promote competition? Would firms be better or worse off if the Commission adopted a "let the buyer beware" policy?

12.8 Your firm sells backup generators to hospitals and clinics. The generators are guaranteed to operate on demand for two years. Your data show that the generators run an average of 42 hours per year. Your firm offers an extended warranty that covers the next three years. Your data show that repairs are needed for 2 percent of units during this three-year period. When repairs are needed, the average cost is $4,000. You charge $400 for the extended warranty, and about 20 percent of your clients buy it.

a. The extended warranty has been a consistent money loser. Claims average $1,000 per customer. How could this be, given the data above?

b. Would raising the premium to $1,000 solve this problem?

c. What would you recommend that your company do to solve this problem?

12.9   For the population as a whole, average spending is $1,190 per year. Those with a family history of cancer (5 percent of the population) spend $20,000 on average, and those with no family history (95 percent of the population) spend $200. An insurer is offering first-dollar coverage for $1,200.

a. You are not risk averse and do not have a family history of cancer. Do you buy coverage?

b. You are not risk averse and have a family history of cancer. Do you buy coverage?

c. If you were risk averse, how would your answers to the two previous questions change?

d. What could an insurer do to prevent this sort of adverse selection?

e. What would be wrong with having everyone undergo a physical exam to qualify for coverage?

12.10 You want to hire a new laboratory technician. Excellent technicians generate $1,000 in value added each week. Adequate technicians generate $500 in value added each week. Half of the graduates are excellent, and half are adequate.

a. You cannot tell who is highly capable and who is adequate. You are prepared to pay each technician his or her value added. What salary do you offer?

b. Who will accept this offer?

c. Is there any way that excellent technicians could communicate their productivity?

d. Propose a compensation system that will attract both types of technicians and pay no one more than his or her value added.

12.11 A new test identifies individuals with a genetic predisposition to heart disease before age 70. People who are predisposed to heart disease cost twice as much to insure as those who are not.

a. Can you make a case that a law prohibiting this test would be a good idea?

b. The test is not expensive. Would you prefer to skip the test and buy insurance at a premium that covers everyone or take the test and buy insurance at a premium that covers your group?

12.12 Your hospital wants to buy practices to expand its primary care networks. You are aware that physicians who want to sell their practices differ. Some love to practice medicine and love seeing patients. They want to sell to focus on patient care 50 hours per week. Some physicians love to play golf and want to provide patient care no more than 35 hours per week. Propose a compensation plan that will allow you to hire only physicians who love to practice.

12.13 Having access to the books and understanding local markets better than new owners, the owners of medical practices generally understand their finances better than prospective buyers do. What sorts of transactions tend to take place as a result of this information asymmetry? Not take place? What can buyers and sellers do to offset this information asymmetry?

12.14 You are considering acquiring Recor, a firm rumored to have developed an effective gene therapy for diabetes. The value of Recor depends on this therapy. If the therapy is effective, Recor is worth $100 per share; otherwise, Recor is worth no more than $20 per share. Your firm's management and marketing strengths should increase the share price by at least 50 percent in either case. You must make an offer for Recor now, before the results of clinical trials are in. The current owner of Recor will sell for the right price. Make an offer for the firm. Explain why you think your offer makes sense.

Chapter Glossary

Agency. An arrangement in which one person (the agent) acts on behalf of another (the principal)

Asymmetric information. Information known to one party in a transaction but not another

Capitation. One payment per person (The payment does not depend on the services provided.)

Case-based payment. One payment for an episode of care (The payment does not change according to the number of services provided.)

Gain sharing. A general strategy for rewarding those who contribute to an organization's success (Profit sharing is one form of gain sharing. Rewards can be based on other criteria as well.)

Opportunism. Taking advantage of a situation without regard for the interests of others

Principal. The organization or individual represented by an agent

Signaling. Sending messages that reveal information another party does not observe

References

Arrow, K. J. 1963. "Uncertainty and the Welfare Economics of Medical Care." *American Economic Review* 53 (5): 941–73.

Bagwell, K., and M. H. Riordan. 1991. "High and Declining Prices Signal Product Quality." *American Economic Review* 81 (1): 224–39.

Baker, G. P., M. C. Jensen, and K. J. Murphy. 1988. "Compensation and Incentives: Practice vs. Theory." *Journal of Finance* 43 (3): 593–616.

Campbell, E. G., R. L. Gruen, J. Mountford, L. G. Miller, P. D. Cleary, and D. Blumenthal. 2007. "A National Survey of Physician–Industry Relationships." *New England Journal of Medicine* 356 (17): 1742–50.

Davis, K., and S. Guterman. 2007. "Rewarding Excellence and Efficiency in Medicare Payments." *Milbank Quarterly* 85 (3): 449–68.

Ginsberg, P., and J. Grossman. 2005. "When the Price Isn't Right: How Inadvertent Payment Incentives Drive Medical Care." *Health Affairs.* [Online article; retrieved 1/15/09.] http://content.healthaffairs.org/cgi/content/full/hlthaff.w5.376/DC1.

Goldfield, N., R. Averill, J. Vertrees, R. Fuller, D. Mesches, G. Moore, J. H. Wasson, and W. Kelly. 2008. "Reforming the Primary Care Physician Payment System." *Journal of Ambulatory Care Management* 31 (1): 24–31.

Josephson, G., and A. Karcz. 1997. "The Impact of Physician Economic Incentives on Admission Rates." *American Journal of Managed Care* 3 (1): 49–56.

Ketcham, J., and M. Furukawa. 2008. "Hospital–Physician Gainsharing in Cardiology." *Health Affairs* 27 (3): 803–12.

Leary, R., and D. Farley. 2005. "Health Plans Slow to Adopt Outpatient Prospective Payment." *Managed Care* 14 (1): 45–52.

Puelz, R., and A. Snow. 1997. "Optimal Incentive Contracting with *Ex Ante* and *Ex Post* Moral Hazards: Theory and Evidence." *Journal of Risk and Uncertainty* 14: 169–88.

Rizzo, J. A., and D. Blumenthal. 1994. "Physician Labor Supply: Do Income Effects Matter?" *Journal of Health Economics* 13 (4): 433–53.

Robinson, J., S. Shortell, R. Li, L. Casalino, and T. Rundall. 2004. "The Alignment and Blending of Payment Incentives Within Physician Organizations." *Health Services Research* 39 (5): 1589–606.

Terry, K. 2007. "Capitation: Still a Factor for Some." *Medical Economics* 84 (23): 38–41.

Trisolini, M., J. Aggarwal, M. Leung, G. Pope, and J. Kautter. 2008. "The Medicare Physician Group Practice Demonstration: Lessons Learned on Improving Quality and Efficiency in Health Care." [Online information; retrieved 5/18/08.] www.commonwealthfund.org/publications.

Weiner, J .P., A. M. Tucker, A. M. Collins, H. Fakhraei, R. Lieberman, C. Abrams, G. R. Trapnell, and J. G. Folkemer. 1998. "The Development of a Risk-Adjusted Capitation Payment System: The Maryland Medicaid Model." *Journal of Ambulatory Care Management* 21 (4): 29–52.

ECONOMIC ANALYSIS OF CLINICAL AND MANAGERIAL INTERVENTIONS

Learning Objectives

After reading this chapter, students will be able to:

- **identify** when a cost-minimization analysis is appropriate,
- **distinguish between** cost-benefit analysis and cost-utility analysis,
- **explain** why economic evaluation is necessary in healthcare, and
- **discuss** the importance of comparing the best alternatives.

Key Concepts

- Analyses of interventions are designed to support decisions, not make them.
- Comparing the most plausible alternatives is vital. Well-done analyses will not be enlightening if we consider the wrong choices.
- Four types of analysis are common: *cost-minimization analysis* (CMA), *cost-effectiveness analysis* (CEA), *cost-utility analysis* (CUA), and *cost-benefit analysis* (CBA).
- The simplest and most productive type of analysis is CMA.
- CBA and CUA are potentially more powerful but pose many questions.
- Modeling costs entails identifying the perspective involved, the resources used, and the opportunity costs of those resources.
- It is best to focus on the direct costs of interventions.
- Modeling benefits is the most difficult part of economic evaluation of clinical interventions.

13.1 Introduction

Until recently, economic analyses of clinical interventions were uncommon. Healthcare decision makers had little or no incentive to assess whether procedures were worth their costs, or even whether those procedures could be done more efficiently. A fee-for-service payment system tells decision makers what procedures are worth. Practical managers in a fee-for-service environment will not worry about genuinely balancing value and cost.

The emergence of global payment systems and the growth of capitation have made economic analyses of clinical interventions more relevant. In a global payment system, getting the same outcome at lower cost directly increases profits. In a capitated system, the options are even greater: Getting the same outcome more cheaply still increases profits, but strategies such as increasing prevention, self-care, or adherence to clinically effective protocols can also have a significant payoff. In short, the value of analyzing clinical interventions has risen sharply.

Analyses of clinical interventions ask deceptively simple questions, such as "Are the benefits of this intervention greater than its costs?" and "Is this intervention better than the alternatives?" Such questions are often difficult to answer, because assessing the benefits of clinical interventions is difficult. While the second question may sound much like the first, it is easier to answer because it does not require assigning the benefits an explicit value.

These questions must be asked, because even in a wealthy society, resources are limited. When an individual chooses to purchase a drug or be screened for a condition, he cannot use those resources for other purposes. The same is true for society. If money spent on an EKG could be used to greater benefit elsewhere, the resources should be reallocated to those other uses. Ideally, we would like to use resources to maximum benefit. Practically, we seek to avoid pure waste and interventions in which the benefits are smaller than the costs.

Why are economic analyses of clinical interventions needed? Public and private insurers need information on which to base coverage decisions. Most patients lack opportunities to become familiar with all the potential outcomes of therapy. In addition, healthcare providers often need information to make the case for a new form of treatment. Because the stakes can be high, patients and providers are reluctant to innovate without evidence.

Analyses of clinical interventions are designed to support decision making, not to make decisions. By providing a framework for synthesizing and understanding information, economic analyses can help decision makers avoid bad decisions.

Four types of analysis are common. Cost-minimization analysis (CMA), cost-effectiveness analysis (CEA), cost-utility analysis (CUA), and cost-benefit analysis (CBA) all compare the costs and benefits of alternative interventions. All four use the same methods to measure costs, but they use different strategies for assessing benefits.

CMA is the most useful for managers. Although it is more limited in scope than the others, it is simpler to apply. CMA answers our second question, "Is this intervention better than the alternatives?" Unfortunately, it cannot answer it in every case. If the better alternative also costs more or if the least expensive alternative does not work as well, CMA is not helpful.

CEA extends CMA somewhat. When the better strategy costs more, CEA answers the question, "What is the cost per unit of this gain?" This simple piece of information is likely to be of genuine value to managers, as it will validate strategies with a small cost per unit and negate those with a large cost per unit. CEA does not, however, directly compare the costs and benefits of a strategy as CUA and CBA do, so it is still a limited tool.

13.2 Cost Analysis

Before examining these four types of analysis in more detail, we will briefly review the basics of cost analysis. Measuring costs involves three tasks:

1. identifying the perspective involved,
2. identifying the resources used, and
3. identifying the opportunity costs of those resources.

Costs are often poorly understood (and poorly measured), even though the issues are seldom very complex.

13.2.1 Identifying Cost Perspective

Identifying a cost perspective is an essential first step. Confusion about costs usually arises because the analyst has not been clear about his perspective. Decision makers usually respond to the costs they see, and different decision makers typically see different portions of the cost. This may seem like an abstract notion, so here is a simple example. An insurance plan (an HMO) wishes to increase use of a generic drug over the brand-name equivalent. The generic product costs a total of $50, of which $4 is paid by the patient and $46 is paid by the plan. The branded product costs a total of $100, of which $5 is paid by the patient and $95 is paid by the plan. From the plan's perspective, switching to the generic saves $49. From the consumer's perspective, switching to the generic saves $1. From the perspective of society as a whole, switching to the generic saves $50. These different perspectives are all valid, yet they may lead to very different choices.

Another example shows how differences in cost perspectives can lead to different perceptions of the cost of a good or service. Suppose the same HMO encourages use of an over-the-counter drug because it is not a covered benefit. The over-the-counter product costs a total of $10, of which $0 is paid by the plan. The prescription product costs a total of $15, of which $5 is paid by the patient and $10 is paid by the plan. From the consumer's perspective, the switch increases costs from $5 to $10. Because consumers share the costs of covered medications with many other beneficiaries, they will want to switch to over-the-counter medications only if they are more effective or more convenient than prescription medications. From the insurer's perspective, the switch reduces costs from $10 to $0. The switch makes sense for the insurer as long as the prescription medication is not "too much better" than the over-the-counter medications. From the perspective of society, the switch reduces costs from $15 to $10 and makes sense only if the over-the-counter medication is "nearly as good" as the prescription medication.

A *societal perspective* on costs is usually the right perspective for two reasons. The societal perspective recognizes all costs, no matter to whom they accrue. Other perspectives typically fail to consider important costs, which is seldom a good long-run strategy. Those to whom costs have been shifted try to avoid them and try to avoid contracting with organizations that shift costs to them.

13.2.2 Identifying Resources and Opportunity Costs

Cost equals the volume of resources used in an activity multiplied by the opportunity cost of those resources. It is useful to keep these two components of cost separate, because either can vary. A clinical understanding of a process makes it easy to identify the resources used in an intervention; a well-documented clinical pathway makes it easier still.

Most of the time the opportunity cost of a resource simply equals what you paid for it. The opportunity cost of $100 in supplies is $100. The opportunity cost of an hour of nursing time is $27 if the total compensation of a nurse is $27 per hour. Calculating the opportunity cost is more complex when the cost of a resource has changed since you bought it and you would not buy it at its current price. In these cases you have to calculate the value of the resource in its best alternative use.

Economic theory provides a powerful tool for simplifying cost analyses. It says, "Focus on the resources you add (or do not need) as a result of this intervention." In other words, "Focus on incremental costs." Even this can be difficult, but it need not be as complex as pondering exactly what proportion of the CFO's compensation should be allocated to a triage process in the emergency room.

13.2.3 Direct and Indirect Costs

Implicit in this advice is a recommendation to focus on the direct costs of interventions, or those costs that result because an intervention has been tried. For example, the costs of a drug and its administration are direct costs of drug therapy. The costs of associated inpatient and outpatient care are also direct costs. If there are healthcare costs associated with ineffectiveness or adverse outcomes, those should be counted as well. By the same token, costs the patient incurs because he or she undertakes this treatment are direct costs. Added childcare, transportation, and dietary costs that result directly from therapy should be counted from a social cost perspective. From the perspective of the healthcare system, however, these added costs for patients would not be counted. (Of course, as we noted above, a cost perspective that ignores the effects on customers is likely to result in poor decisions.)

Most "indirect" costs represent a confusion of costs with benefits. Healthier people typically spend more on food, recreation, entertainment, and other joys of life, but this additional spending is not a part of the costs of interventions that restored health. (Individuals have independently made the judgment that this additional spending is worth it.) By the same token we should not treat a recovered patient's future spending as a cost of the intervention that permitted her recovery—unless, as with transplant patients' immunosuppressive drugs, these costs are an integral part of the intervention. That a transplant patient feels healthy enough to play tennis certainly signals that her operation was a success, but the cost of knee surgery for this overenthusiastic athlete should not be reckoned as a cost of the transplant.

13.3 Types of Analysis

We have identified four types of analysis: CBA, CEA, CUA, and CMA. Be aware that mislabeling is the norm, not the exception. A "cost-benefit analysis" could be anything, and the meaning of "cost-effectiveness analysis" has changed over the years. Figure 13.1 shows when each is needed.

If it is really difficult to decide which strategy is best, it shouldn't matter, since they all support decision making. If the options look so similar

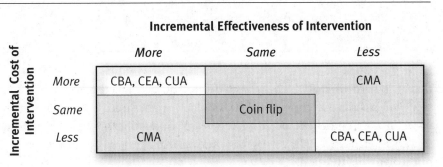

FIGURE 13.1

Using Decision-Support Tools

Case 13.1 **Teledermatology**

"Well, this does not suggest to me that it makes sense to push ahead with fancy telemedicine equipment for our practice. As I read the data, it costs us $280 to provide a consult to a patient via telemedicine and $320 to do it face-to-face. It might boost our profits a little, but I can't imagine too many patients will want to give up meeting their dermatologist in person. So," our CFO summed up, "I recommend against this project."

"If that were the whole story," said Kim Jarrett, "I would agree with you. But this looks only at our costs. We need to think about the costs patients bear. Many of our patients are children, so they have to be driven across town by a parent. By the time you figure in the travel costs and time costs parents incur to bring their children here, a face-to-face visit could easily cost $100 more than a telemedicine visit. And that back-of-the-envelope calculation just looks at people in the local area. We know children in the western half of the state are not getting the care they should. There are very few dermatologists out there, and there are no dermatologists who specialize in treating pediatric skin cancer. The time and travel costs for those patients could easily be $200 per visit. We can't just look at our own costs."

"I hadn't thought of that," said Carroll Briggs. "I was focusing on these cost estimates, not taking into account the opportunity to do group visits—which our patients have been asking about—very inexpensively. This technology will let one of our doctors or nurses talk to eight patients at once in their homes. It's mostly teaching and coaching, so the patients do not need ultra-high-resolution monitors on their home computers. We could even do some follow-up visits that way, so I think there are options this analysis of $280 per visit does not consider."

Discussion questions:
- Does Kim's point about patients' costs make sense?
- Which perspective on costs looks more like a societal perspective to you?
- Would using telemedicine equipment mean completely giving up face-to-face meetings with a dermatologist?
- What would be the advantage, if any, of being able to serve patients in the western half of the state?
- What would be the advantage, if any, of being able to offer telemedicine group visits?
- What is your assessment of the promise of telemedicine for this practice?

---

that it is hard to say which is best, do not do a detailed analysis. A "coin flip" will suffice. Of course, when populations are large, even small differences in cost or benefit per case can result in significant differences from society's perspective. However, for working managers, small differences are not worthy of attention.

Sidebar 13.1 Steps in CMA

1. Estimate the expected costs for each option.
2. Show that the least-cost option has outcomes at least as good as higher-cost alternatives.

A CMA Example

Current treatment guidelines for patients hospitalized with community-acquired pneumonia recommend antibiotic therapy for eight days. The scientific basis for eight days of antibiotics is limited, and there are suggestions that briefer treatments may be appropriate. Because community-acquired pneumonia is a common problem, substantial savings might be possible with briefer treatments.

Opmeer et al. (2007) conducted a randomized control trial to compare three-day and eight-day antibiotic therapies. At day three of treatment, patients with community-acquired pneumonia who had significantly improved were randomly assigned to five days of placebo or five days of antibiotics. Patients were then followed for 28 days.

Although patients who received three-day treatment had shorter hospital stays and missed less work, none of the clinical outcomes was significantly different from the outcomes for eight-day treatment. Costs for the three-day treatment were about 4 percent lower.

13.4 CMA: Cost-Minimization Analysis

The simplest and most productive type of analysis is CMA, which identifies the intervention with the lowest costs. As long as the intervention has outcomes at least as good as those of the alternatives, a CMA is the analysis of choice. While CMA avoids most of the problems associated with measuring benefits, it does not escape them entirely. The most common problem in CMA is a lack of evidence that the least-cost option has outcomes at least as good as the other choices.

13.5 CEA: Cost-Effectiveness Analysis

CEA recognizes that it may be useful, when a more effective intervention costs more, to measure the incremental cost of improving outcomes. In at least some cases the incremental cost will be so high or so low that a decision can be based on it. In our detailed example in Sidebar 13.2, CEA estimates the cost per life year saved.

Sidebar 13.2 Steps in CEA

1. Estimate the expected costs for each option.
2. Establish how much the higher-cost option improves outcomes.
3. Calculate the cost per unit of improvement in outcome (e.g., the cost per life year gained or the cost per infection avoided).

A CEA Example

There are many reasons pregnant women should stop smoking, but over 25 percent of low-income women smoke during pregnancy. Trying to increase quit rates, Ruger et al. (2008) conducted a randomized control trial of motivational interviewing by public health nurses for low-income pregnant women. Motivational interviewing is a type of counseling that helps clients explore why they want to stop smoking, what problems smoking causes for them, why they are ambivalent about quitting, and how life as a nonsmoker would be different.

Motivational interviewing did not appear to increase the number of women who quit smoking, but it appeared to help those who had already quit avoid a relapse. Among patients who had recently quit smoking when they entered the study, 82.1 percent of usual care patients and 57.1 percent of motivational interview patients resumed smoking during the six months of follow-up.

Adding motivational interviewing increased costs by $304. It also reduced the probability of a relapse by 25 percentage points and added 0.36 life years. So the incremental cost per relapse prevented was $1,217 and the incremental cost per life year gained was $851. The cost per life year was quite low, suggesting that using motivational interviewing to reduce relapse rates is sensible.

In some cases CEA is not helpful. If the cost per life year saved is $35,000 or if the cost per injury prevented is $10,000, the answer will not seem obvious. In these cases CBA or CUA may be needed.

13.6 CBA: Cost-Benefit Analysis

CBA is also relatively simple, but its validity is unknown. CBA is appropriate when the option with the best outcomes costs more. CBA begins with a comparison of two or more options to find out how their costs differ, then attempts to estimate the difference in benefits directly. There are two very different strategies for estimating benefits. One uses statistical techniques to infer how much consumers are willing to pay to avoid risks. The other uses surveys of the relevant population to determine whether the added benefits are worth the cost.

Neither method's validity has been clearly established. The fundamental challenge arises from concerns about consumers' abilities to make decisions involving small probabilities of harm. If consumers do not assess these probabilities accurately, their life choices and their responses to surveys will not be reliable. In addition, there are always multiple challenges to the validity of statistical inferences, and statistical estimates of benefits are imprecise. Surveys may not give us valid measures of willingness to pay or willingness to accept compensation. First, they ask consumers to make complex assessments of services they have not yet used. Answers to hypothetical, complex questions are suspect. Second, consumers may misrepresent their preferences, believing they will have to pay more out-of-pocket if they answer willingness-to-pay questions accurately. Therefore, even though CBA can provide invaluable information to decision makers, its accuracy can be suspect.

Two other criticisms are worth noting. Early CBA studies based estimates of benefits on estimates of increases in labor market earnings. A few minutes of reflection will reveal problems with this approach. Is improved health for retired persons of no value? If people are willing to pay out-of-pocket for the care of their pets (who have no earning power), aren't changes in earnings a poor guide to the value of medical interventions? Earnings-based estimates of benefits have left a legacy of skepticism of CBA among healthcare analysts. A second complaint is that willingness to pay usually rises with income. This is profoundly troubling to analysts who would prefer a healthcare system that is more egalitarian than the current system in the United States. (While this is not really a criticism of CBA, it is sometimes presented as such.)

To illustrate how CBA works, return to the example of the switch from a branded product to a generic one. Recall that the branded drug cost $100 and the generic cost $50. An uninsured consumer would buy the branded product only if its benefits were large enough for her to be willing to pay $100. Few consumers would be willing to pay this much to get the branded product, because branded and generic products seldom differ. For current users of a branded drug, however, there are both real and perceived risks to switching, such as the risk of an allergic reaction to different inert ingredients. Remember, from the insured consumer's perspective, the cost differential is only $1, from $5 for the branded product to $4 for the generic. Current users of the drug may be willing to pay $75, in which case the marginal benefit of the branded drug will appear larger than its marginal cost. Current users have an incentive to make sure others bear the financial risk of higher costs. Asking people who are not current users is also problematic. The opinion of someone who does not have a disease the drug is intended to treat or has not used both drugs is not likely to hold much value.

Sidebar 13.3 Steps in CBA

1. Estimate the expected incremental costs of the more expensive option.
2. Survey consumers to find out whether they would be (a) willing to pay enough to cover the added costs of an option with better outcomes or (b) willing to accept compensation that would be less than the cost savings of an option with worse outcomes.
3. Or, use market data to estimate how much consumers are willing to pay to avoid risks or willing to accept to take on risks.
4. Compare the incremental benefits and costs.

A CBA Example

Do the benefits of poison control centers exceed their costs? A team from the University of California–San Francisco found that the average respondent was willing to pay just under $6 per month to have access to a poison control center (Phillips et al. 1997). This easily exceeded the cost of providing the services of a poison control center, which averaged less than 10 cents per household per month.

Willingness to pay represents an attractive way of measuring the benefits of a service like a poison control center. First and foremost, both the caller and the victim typically benefit from the service. Even if the caller knows the victim only casually, it seems likely that she would be willing to pay something to reduce the stress and anxiety associated with a poisoning. Second, most of the benefits of a poison control center are intangible. Few poisonings result in serious injury or death, and most can be treated at home. Third, people may be willing to pay a little just to know that the service is there, even if they are not likely to use it.

13.7 CUA: Cost-Utility Analysis

CUA rivals CBA as a complete comparison of alternative interventions (note that a number of analysts do not distinguish between CEA and CUA). CUA seeks to measure consumer values by eliciting valuations of health states. This information is then used to "quality adjust" health gains, so that decision makers can consider the cost per quality-adjusted life year (QALY) saved (we will explain how QALYs are calculated later).

CUA is complex and its validity is unknown. It is appropriate whenever CBA is, and at a formal level the two are essentially equivalent. At a practical level, however, the process of calculating benefits is different. CUA measures how alternative interventions change the health status of patients and how patients evaluate those changes.

The team elicited this information via a telephone survey of Bay Area residents. The sample included three groups. One group consisted of residents who had tried to call but had been blocked from using the local poison control center because their county government refused to contribute its share of the budget. Less than 1 percent of this group was unwilling to pay anything for access. Another group consisted of residents who had called the poison control center. Again, under 1 percent of this group was unwilling to pay anything for access. A third group consisted of residents who had never called the poison control center, of which 20 percent was unwilling to pay anything for access.

Surveyors elicited willingness-to-pay data via a bidding process. They asked respondents whether they would be willing to pay a randomly chosen amount per month for access to the center. If the respondent said no, the surveyor countered with a lower number. If the respondent said, yes, the surveyor countered with a higher number.

Although the simplicity and power of these results demonstrates some of the attractions of a CBA, this study also points out some of the associated pitfalls. Responses were significantly influenced by the initial willingness to pay what surveyors suggested to them. The possibility that the interviewers, who already had an answer in mind, biased the study's results cannot be ruled out. In addition, the interviewers did not offer alternative uses of funds or get respondents to rank types of spending. Some studies have found that focusing on one service tends to inflate respondents' willingness to pay. Fundamentally, we still do not know how valid respondents' answers are, although it seems unlikely that the conclusions of this study are totally incorrect, given that willingness to pay was 50 times cost.

Figure 13.2 walks through the calculations for a CUA. Suppose 215 people each get treatments A and B. At the end of one year the number of survivors differs for the two treatments (N_A and N_B), as does the average utility level (U_A and U_B). We use these data to calculate how many additional QALYs we get as a result of using treatment B. We then calculate the cost per QALY if we switch to treatment B.

Four uncertainties are associated with this calculation, aside from the usual problems assessing the clinical effectiveness of treatments. First, should we limit our questions to patients? Family, friends, and strangers are sometimes willing to help patients afford care. Second, can patients answer our questions about satisfaction adequately and accurately? Third, what discount rate should we use? While the example uses 3 percent, another rate might give us different answers, and we do not know what

			QALY$_A$			QALY$_B$	QALY$_B$ – QALY$_A$	
							Discounted	
	N_A	U_A	$N_A \times U_A$	N_B	U_B	$N_B \times U_B$	*0%*	*3%*
Year 1 outcomes	200	0.95	190.00	210	0.96	201.60	11.60	11.26
Year 2 outcomes	195	0.94	183.30	199	0.93	185.07	1.77	1.67
							13.37	12.93
Cost per QALY (with a $300,000 cost difference between A and B)							$22,438	$23,201

NOTE: N$_A$ and N$_B$ refer to the number of participants. U$_A$ and U$_B$ refer to the average utility score of participants.

FIGURE 13.2
A Cost-Utility
Analysis

the right rate is. Fourth, assuming all other calculations are correct, at what cost per QALY should we draw the line? At the risk of sounding unduly negative, the validity of CUA hinges on finding satisfactory answers to these questions, which is not likely.

Unlike CMA or CBA, CUA requires that the analyst explicitly discount future QALYs. A technique commonly used in banking and finance, *discounting* reflects benefits we realize far in the future being worth less than benefits we realize now. This is true because money can earn interest. To pay a bill that will come due in the future, one can set aside a smaller amount today. For example, if we invest $100 at an interest rate of 7 percent, we will have $160.58 at the end of ten years. We can reverse this calculation to show that the value of a guaranteed payment of $160.58 that we will get in ten years is $100.

As long as the interest rate is fixed, discounting is easy to figure on a spreadsheet. A single formula, $PV \times (1 + r)^n = FV$, lets us do all the necessary calculations. In this formula, PV refers to the "present value" of future costs or benefits, or the amount we are investing today; r refers to the interest rate; n refers to the number of time periods involved; and FV refers to the "future value" of future costs or benefits, or the amount we will have at the end of our investment. We use the same formula to calculate the present value of future costs and benefits. The formula now becomes $PV = FV/(1 + r)^n$. If we knew the size and timing of an intervention's costs and benefits and the right discount rate, calculating the present value of the QALYs associated with it would be a simple matter. In fact, we don't know the right discount rate and are not sure the discount rate is constant for a given individual, let alone for different individuals. Sensitivity analysis is the best we can do in this regard. This entails varying the discount rate over a "reasonable" range (typically 0 to 10 percent) and seeing if the answer changes. If not, the result is insensitive to the value of the discount rate. But if the answer does change, we have to use our judgment.

Sidebar 13.4 Steps in CUA

1. Estimate the expected costs for each option.
2. Estimate the number of people alive in each year in each cohort.
3. Using a survey of consumers, estimate the average utility score for each option for each person who is alive in each year.
4. Multiply the utility score (which will range from zero to one) by the number of people alive in each year for all the cohorts being compared. The product is the number of quality-adjusted life years (QALYs) for each cohort.
5. Discount the QALYs using rates of 2 to 5 percent.
6. Add the QALYs for each option, then find the difference.
7. Divide the difference in cost between options by the difference in QALYs.
8. Decide whether the cost per QALY is too high.

A CUA Example

Are automobile air bags cost-effective? A highly skilled team from the Harvard Center for Risk Analysis studied this question and concluded that the answer depended heavily on the location of the air bag (Graham et al. 1997). This study confronted the difficult issues posed by discounting and quality adjustment. The benefits of the study extend over a long period of time, and the authors chose to examine the cost per QALY, rather than the cost per death avoided.

The team began with baseline data about accidents, fatalities, nonfatal injuries, and seat belt use. They used this information to calculate the net number of deaths and injuries that would be avoided by use of air bags. (They looked at net deaths because, especially for infants, children, and very small adults, air bags can cause death in accidents that would not usually result in death.)

The team concluded that the incremental cost of equipping 10 million vehicles with *driver's side* air bags would be $2.21 billion. They estimated that doing so would save 93,106 QALYs. As a result, the incremental cost-effectiveness ratio is just under $24,000 per QALY. At $1.33 billion the incremental cost of equipping 10 million vehicles with *passenger's side* air bags is substantially less. But, largely because front passenger seats are often unoccupied, the incremental effectiveness of air bags is much smaller. The team estimated that adding passenger's side air bags would save just 21,796 QALYs, meaning that the incremental cost per QALY was $61,000. Because innovations are cost-effective if the cost per QALY is less than $50,000 and clearly not cost-effective if the cost per QALY is more than $100,000, passenger's side air bags are of uncertain value. There is strong support for the premise that the value of driver's side air bags exceeds their cost, as consumers in Asia and Europe are buying air bags voluntarily. Of course the inability of CUA to determine whether passenger's side air bags are a good value or not is a shortcoming.

(continued)

Sidebar 13.4 continued

The study conducts a full-scale sensitivity analysis, in which the driver's side air bag remains cost-effective. Some of the changes in parameter push passenger's side air bags toward the cut-off point. For example, at the lower end of the effectiveness assumptions, the cost per QALY for passenger's side air bags exceeds $100,000.

Many technical issues remain to be resolved in CUA. This study includes the net change in healthcare costs in the cost of air bags. This is controversial. We would argue that although a reduction in injuries is a benefit, this confuses two very separate decisions—whether to install air bags and how much medical care to seek in the case of crash-related injuries. Others would disagree. As always, the validity of the quality adjustment that underlies the construction of QALYs is unknown.

The real challenge, however, is to identify the options to which mandating air bags should be compared. For example, only when compared with stricter enforcement of seat belt laws or vigorous educational campaigns to encourage seat belt use can we really assess whether mandatory passenger's air bags are cost-effective.

13.8 Conclusion

Except for CMA or possibly CEA, our advice is, "Don't try this at home." When you need evidence to make a decision, turn to the literature. If no guidance is to be found there, do a CMA or CEA (or modify existing studies using your costs). If these tools do not provide a clear direction, use clinical judgment. CBA and CUA are research tools, not management tools.

Still, these techniques can help make your organization more efficient. Applied judiciously, they will help your organization identify and provide the most efficient therapies, which will reduce your costs and increase your options.

The importance of comparing the right options is often lost in the discussion of these analyses. Failing to compare reasonable alternatives renders CMA, CEA, CBA, and CUA useless. The best choice will usually be clear if the most plausible alternatives are compared. And if the best choice is not clear, either choice may be appropriate.

Homework

13.1   Why have economic analyses of clinical and administrative innovations become more important?

13.2   Why is cost minimization analysis most likely to be useful for managers?

13.3   Why would an economist object to including overhead costs in a CMA analysis?

13.4   A clinic finds that by eliminating appointments it can reduce costs. The clinic is able to eliminate some telephone staff, and physicians become more productive. Patients wait until the physician is available, so there is virtually no down time. Does this analysis adopt a societal view of costs? Why might this analysis result in a bad managerial decision?

13.5   Treating a patient with congestive heart failure with tPlex rather than Isother increases average life expectancy to 12.3 years from 11.5 years. The added cost of therapy is $14,000. What is the cost per life year? Should you choose tPlex or Isother?

13.6   Compared with a drip system, a new type of infusion pump reduces the cost of administering chemotherapy from $25 per dose to $20 per dose. The complication rate of each system is 2 percent. Which should you choose? What sort of analysis should you do?

13.7   After making your choice in the previous problem, you discover an infusion pump with a dosage monitoring system costs $15 per dose. Its monitoring functions reduce the complication rate to 1 percent. Which of the three options do you prefer? What principle does this illustrate?

13.8   Switching from one anesthesia drug to another reduces costs by $100 per patient. What additional information do you need to do a cost-minimization analysis?

13.9   A vaccine costs $200 per patient. Administration of the vaccine to 1,000 people is expected to increase the number of pain-free days for this population from 360,000 to 362,000. Calculate the cost per additional pain-free day due to vaccination. Is this a good investment?

13.10   An acute care hospital has found that having geriatric nurse specialists take charge of discharge planning for stroke patients reduces length of stay from 5.4 days to 5.2 days. On average the geriatric nurse specialist (who earns $27 per hour including fringes) spends 3.3 hours on discharge planning per patient. Supply and telephone costs are less than $10 per discharge plan. Your accounting staff tell you the average cost per day is $860 and the incremental cost per day is about $340. Is this a financially attractive innovation? Whether it is or not, what alternatives should the hospital consider?

13.11   The current cost function for a lab that evaluates Pap smears is $C = 200,000 + 25 \times Q$. Q, the annual volume of tests, is forecast to be 30,000. Incremental cost is $25 because each evaluation requires $20 worth of a technician's time and $5 worth of supplies. Calculate the average cost of an evaluation.

13.12 You are comparing replacing the current lab, which has a cost function of C = 200,000 + 25 × Q with an automated lab that has a cost function of C = 300,000 + 20 × Q. Doing so would reduce the error rate from 1.5 percent to 1 percent. Your volume is expected to be 18,000 tests per year. Should you choose the automated lab? Briefly explain your logic.

13.13 The expected cost of Betazine therapy is $544. It is effective 57 percent of the time, with a 6 percent chance of an adverse drug reaction. Below are data for Alphazine, a new treatment. Estimate the rate of adverse drug reaction and the expected cost of treatment. Use Excel to construct a decision tree for this problem. Should you choose Alphazine or Betazine?

			Probability	Cost
Effective	63%	Adverse drug reaction	5%	$700
		No adverse drug reaction	95%	$500
Ineffective	37%	Adverse drug reaction	5%	$800
		No adverse drug reaction	95%	$600

Chapter Glossary

Cost-benefit analysis. An analysis that compares the value of an innovation with its costs. Value is measured as willingness to pay for the innovation or willingness to accept compensation to allow it to be implemented.

Cost-effectiveness analysis. An analysis that measures the cost of an innovation per unit of change in a single outcome.

Cost-minimization analysis. An analysis that measures the cost of two or more innovations with the same patient outcomes.

Cost-utility analysis. An analysis that measures the cost of an innovation per quality-adjusted life year.

Discounting. Adjusting the value of future costs and benefits to reflect the willingness of consumers to trade current consumption for future consumption. Usually future values are discounted by $1/(1 + r)^n$, with r the discount rate and n the number of periods in the future the cost or benefit will be realized.

Societal perspective. A perspective that takes account of all costs and benefits, no matter to whom they accrue.

References

Graham, J. D., K. M. Thompson, S. J. Goldie, M. Segui-Gomez, and M. C. Weinstein. 1997. "The Cost-Effectiveness of Air Bags by Seating Position." *Journal of the American Medical Association* 278 (17): 1418–24.

Opmeer, B. C., R. el Moussaoui, P. M. M. Bossuyt, P. Speelman, J. M. Prins, and C. A. J. M. de Borgie. 2007. "Costs Associated with Shorter Duration of Antibiotic Therapy in Hospitalized Patients with Mild-to-Moderate-Severe Community-Acquired Pneumonia." *Journal of Antimicrobial Chemotherapy* 60 (5): 1131–36.

Phillips, K. A., R. K. Homan, H. S. Luft, D. H. Hiatt, D. R. Olson, T. E. Kearney, and S. E. Heard. 1997. "Willingness to Pay for Poison Control Centers." *Journal of Health Economics* 16 (3): 343–57.

Ruger, J. P., M. C. Weinstein, S. K. Hammond, M. H. Kearney, and K. M. Emmons. 2008. "Cost-Effectiveness of Motivational Interviewing for Smoking Cessation and Relapse Prevention Among Low-Income Pregnant Women: A Randomized Controlled Trial." *Value in Health* 11 (2): 191–98.

Suver, J., S. R. Arikian, J. J. Doyle, S. W. Sweeney, and M. Hagan. 1995. "Use of Anesthesia Selection in Controlling Surgery Costs in an HMO Hospital." *Clinical Therapeutics* 17 (3): 561–71.

14

PROFITS, MARKET STRUCTURE, AND MARKET POWER

After reading this chapter, students will be able to:

- **describe** standard models of market structure,
- **discuss** the importance of market power in healthcare,
- **calculate** the impact of market share on pricing,
- **apply** Porter's model to pricing, and
- **discuss** the determinants of market structure.

Key Concepts

- If the demand for its products is not perfectly elastic, a firm has some market power.
- Most healthcare organizations have some market power because their rivals' products are not perfect substitutes.
- Having fewer rivals increases market power.
- Firms with no rivals are called *monopolists*.
- Firms with only a few rivals are called *oligopolists*.
- More market power allows larger markups over marginal cost.
- Barriers to entry increase market power.
- Regulation is often a source of market power.
- Product differentiation and advertising can be sources of market power.

14.1 Introduction

What distinguishes very competitive markets (those with below-average profit margins) from less competitive markets (those with above-average profit margins)? An influential analysis by Michael E. Porter (1985) argues that profitability depends on five factors:

1. the nature of rivalry among existing firms,
2. the risk of entry by potential rivals,
3. the bargaining power of customers,
4. the bargaining power of suppliers, and
5. the threat from substitute products.

For the most part, Porter's model explains profit variations in terms of variations in market power. Firms in industries with muted price competition, little risk of entry by rivals, limited customer bargaining power, and few satisfactory substitutes have significant market power. Firms with market power face customer demands that are not particularly price elastic. As a result, markups can be large. We will use the Porter framework to examine the links between profits, market structure, and market power.

Three characteristics of healthcare markets reduce their competitiveness. First, many healthcare markets have only a few competitors, which mutes rivalry among firms. Second, this muted rivalry persists in many healthcare markets because cost and regulatory barriers limit entry. Third, there are few close substitutes for many healthcare products. This makes the market demand less elastic and may make the demand for an individual firm's products less elastic. These factors give healthcare firms market power and allow high markups.

The bargaining power of suppliers varies. A detailed examination of differences in suppliers' bargaining power is beyond the scope of this book, but one change is important to note. Physicians are suppliers to many healthcare organizations, and physicians' incomes have stagnated since the early 1990s, causing deterioration of their bargaining position.

The most significant change in healthcare markets has been the growth of managed care. Managed care dramatically enhances the bargaining power of most healthcare customers. As a result, many healthcare firms face more competitive markets and narrower margins than they previously faced.

Profit-oriented managers will usually seek to gain market power. The most ambitious will try to change the nature of competition. For example, faced with determined managed care negotiators, healthcare providers may merge to reduce costs and improve their bargaining positions, which can improve margins. But even when an organization cannot change a market's competitive structure, it still has two options: It can seek to become the low-cost producer, or it can seek to differentiate its products from those of the competition. Either strategy can boost margins, even in competitive markets.

14.2 Rivalry Among Existing Firms

Most healthcare organizations have some market power. Price elasticities of demand are small enough that an organization will not lose all its business to rivals with slightly lower prices. Market power has several implications. Obviously, it means firms have some discretion on pricing, since the market does not dictate what they will charge. Flexibility in pricing and product specifications means managers must consider a broad range of strategies, including how to compete. Some markets have aggressive competition in price and product innovation; other markets do not. Managers have to decide what strategy best fits their circumstances. The prospect of market power also gives healthcare organizations a strong incentive to differentiate their products. The amount of market power an organization has typically depends on how much its products differ from competitors' in terms of quality, convenience, or some other attribute.

Healthcare organizations generally have market power because their competitors' products are imperfect substitutes. Reasons for this include differences in location or other attributes, or even product familiarity. For example, a pharmacy across town is less convenient than one nearby, even if it has lower prices. Because consumers choose to patronize the more expensive but closer pharmacy, it has market power.

Medical goods and services are typically "experience" products, in that consumers must use a product to ascertain that it offers better value than another. For instance, a patient will not know whether a new dentist will meet her needs until her first visit. Likewise, consumers will have to try a generic drug to be sure it works as well as the branded version. Because of this need to try out healthcare products, comparison of medical goods and services is costly, and consumers tend not to change products when price differences are small. These factors make it difficult to assess whether competing products are good substitutes, thus increasing market power.

As we will see in section 14.7, advertising decisions depend on the differences that determine market power. Attribute-based differences usually demand extensive advertising. Information-based differences often reward restrictions on advertising.

Many healthcare providers have few competitors. This is true for hospitals and nursing homes in most markets, and often for rural physicians. Where the market is small, either because the population is small or because the service is highly specialized, competitors will usually be few. And when there are few rivals, all have some market power, if only because each controls a significant share of the market. Firms with few competitors recognize that they have flexibility in pricing and that what their rivals do will affect them.

Sidebar 14.1 Do Physicians Really Have Market Power?

It appears they do, even though there are many physicians in most markets. Two studies have attempted to calculate the price elasticity of demand faced by individual physicians (Lee and Hadley 1981; McCarthy 1985). One estimated price elasticities from −2.8 to −5.1; another found a very similar range of −3.1 to −3.3. Not surprisingly, demand for the services of individual physicians is much more elastic than the demand for physicians' services as a whole. (After all, other physicians may not be perfect substitutes for your physician, but they are fairly close substitutes.) These estimates suggest markups will be large, meaning physicians have a good deal of market power. Furthermore, by organizing themselves into independent practice associations, which bargain with insurers on behalf of member physicians, physicians effectively increase their market share and market power (Page 2004).

A perfectly competitive market, in which buyers and sellers are price takers (i.e., a market in which both believe that they cannot alter the market price), offers a baseline with which to contrast other market structures. In perfect competition, firms operate under the assumption that demand is very price-elastic. The only way to realize above-normal profits is to be more efficient than the competition. Firms disregard the actions of their rivals, in part because potential entrants face no barriers and in part because there are so many rivals. In any other market structure, organizations will produce less and charge higher prices.

Few healthcare markets even remotely resemble perfectly competitive markets. Some have only one supplier and are said to be *monopolistic*. For example, the only pharmacist in town has a monopoly. A number of markets have many rivals, all claiming a small share of the market. At first glance these markets may look perfectly competitive, but there is one key difference: Customers do not view the services of one supplier as perfect substitutes for the services of another. Each dentist has a different location, a different personality, or a different treatment style. Markets such as these are said to be *monopolistically competitive*.

Other markets have only a few competitors. These markets are said to be *oligopolistic*. Markets with many competitors can also be oligopolistic if a few competitors have a significant market share. A local market with two hospitals serving the same area is oligopolistic, as is a PPO market with 15 firms, the two largest firms of which have 40 percent of the market. Because the decisions of some competitors determine the strategies of others, oligopolistic markets differ from other markets in an important way. Oligopolists must act strategically and recognize their mutual interdependence. We will explore this in more detail in Chapter 15.

14.3 Customers' Bargaining Power

A longtime distinguishing feature of healthcare markets is that there are many buyers, all with limited bargaining power. This is not true of every market. The emergence of managed care firms, which identify efficient providers and those who will give substantial price concessions, changes the picture. (Of course, Medicare and Medicaid, the original PPOs, have had a major influence on healthcare markets since their inception.) So in addition to the number of sellers, healthcare market structures depend on the market shares of PPOs and HMOs (including Medicare and Medicaid, where appropriate) and the number of each in the market.

14.4 Entry by Potential Rivals

Barriers to entry in healthcare markets may be market-based or regulation-based. Generally, regulation-based barriers are more effective. Whatever the source, restrictions on entry reduce the number of competing providers and make demand less price elastic. In other words, entry restrictions, whether necessary or not, increase market power.

The best way to erect entry barriers and gain market power is to have the government do it for you. This strategy has two fundamental advantages. First, it is perfectly legal and eliminates public and private suits alleging anti-trust violations. Second, the resulting market power is usually more permanent, because government-sanctioned entry barriers will not be eroded by market competition.

State licensure forms much of the basis for market power in healthcare. Licensure prevents entry by suppliers with similar qualifications and encroachments by suppliers with lesser qualifications. For example, state licensure laws typically require that pharmacy technicians work under the direct supervision of registered pharmacists and that a registered pharmacist supervise no more than two technicians. These restrictions clearly protect pharmacists' jobs by limiting competition from technicians.

Intellectual property rights can also provide entry barriers. Innovating organizations can establish a monopoly for a limited period by securing patents. A U.S. patent gives the holder a monopoly for 17 years. The patent holder must disclose the details of the new product or process in the application but is free to exploit the patent and sell or license the rights. Patents are vitally important in the pharmaceutical industry, as generic products are excluded from the market until the patent expires.

Copyrights also create monopolies that protect intellectual property rights. Unlike patents, copyrights protect only a particular expression of an idea, not the idea itself. Copyright monopolies normally last for the life of

---

Sidebar 14.2 Managed Care Affects Rivalry

The expansion of managed care changed the nature of rivalry in competitive healthcare markets. HMO and PPO plans have been most successful in markets with keen competition among hospitals. Bamezai and colleagues (1999) found that hospital costs grew more slowly in markets with high HMO or PPO penetration than in markets with low penetration. However, even in markets with many competing hospitals, cost growth has not slowed unless managed care has successfully penetrated the market.

The study also concluded that HMOs did more to control costs than did PPOs. In competitive, high-HMO markets, costs rose more slowly than in competitive, high-PPO markets. HMOs usually build smaller provider networks than PPOs, so HMOs can bargain more effectively than PPOs can. In addition, HMOs make more use of capitation and case rates, giving hospitals and physicians much stronger incentives to control costs.

These results are consistent with recent trends. As HMOs have lost market share and hospitals have consolidated, the ability of private insurers to control costs has eroded.

---

the author plus 50 years. Trademarks (distinctive visual images that belong to a particular organization) also grant monopoly rights. As long as they are used and defended, trademarks never expire. All these legal monopolies create formidable barriers to entry for potential competitors.

Strategic actions can also prevent or slow entry by rivals. Rivals will not want to launch unprofitable ventures, and firms can try to ensure entrants will lose money. Preemption, limit pricing, innovation, and mergers are common tactics. *Preemption* is moving quickly to build excess capacity in a region or product line and thereby ward off entry. For example, building a hospital with excess capacity means a second hospital would face formidable barriers. Not only would it exacerbate the capacity surplus, but this excess capacity could cause a price war. Managed care firms would not miss the opportunity to grab larger discounts. Worse still for the prospective entrant, most of the costs of the established firm are fixed. Its best strategy would be to capture as much of the market as it can by aggressive price cutting. In contrast, the rival's costs are all incremental. It can avoid years of losses by building elsewhere.

Limit pricing is another tactic established firms or those with established products can use. *Limit pricing* is setting prices low enough to discourage potential entrants. By giving up some profits now, an organization

Sidebar 14.3 Mergers Result in Price Increases

Between 2000 and 2006, 980 acute-care hospitals changed hands. Although the pace has slowed since the 1990s, the consolidation of hospital markets continues. In principle, the merger of two hospitals allows cost savings. The merged hospitals would need less excess capacity to cope with spikes in demand, could avoid duplicate services, and could share some overhead expenses. Offsetting this benefit is the difficulty of merging two disparate organizations. In addition, evidence that consolidation reduces costs is mixed (Ferrier and Valdmanis 2004).

It does appear that small hospitals can realize significant cost savings by merging. Dranove (1998) estimates that administrative costs per discharge are 34 percent lower in a 200-bed hospital than in a 100-bed hospital. Overall cost per discharge in nonrevenue cost centers is 24 percent lower in a 200-bed hospital than in a 100-bed hospital. For larger hospitals, size conveys few cost advantages. Cost per discharge in nonrevenue cost centers is only 1 percent lower in a 400-bed hospital than in a 200-bed hospital. The policy of the Federal Trade Commission and the Department of Justice not to challenge mergers if one of the hospitals has fewer than 100 beds appears to be a solid one.

The other motive for consolidation is to increase market power. A single hospital or a two-hospital system is in a much better bargaining position than two independent hospitals serving the same area. An analysis by Capps and Dranove (2004) verified this prediction, concluding that consolidation allowed hospitals to negotiate larger-than-average PPO price increases. Evidence points to increased concentration resulting in higher prices, although reliable data on what hospitals actually get paid is scarce.

Recognizing that hospital consolidations could push prices up, federal antitrust authorities have opposed some hospital mergers. The authorities have lost most of these suits. Courts have generally seen the not-for-profit status of merging hospitals as a guarantee of price restraint, although there is little support for this expectation in the economics literature.

On the contrary, most studies have found that merging not-for-profit hospitals significantly increase markups (Gaynor and Vogt 2003). For example, a study of California hospitals found that mergers among not-for-profit hospitals resulted in price increases ranging from 0.3 to 7.3 percent (Keeler, Melnick, and Zwanziger 1999). The effects of mergers depend on the nature of the hospitals involved and the nature of the competition in their market. The estimates suggest that if two small hospitals in a competitive metropolitan area merge, their ability to negotiate higher prices will be limited. In contrast, if two large hospitals in a smaller town merge, their ability to negotiate can be substantial.

can avoid the even bigger profit reductions competition might cause later. In essence, the firm acts as though demand were more elastic than it is. Limit pricing only works if the firm is an aggressive innovator. Otherwise, competitors will eventually enter the market with lower costs or better quality, and the payoff to limit pricing will be minimal.

Innovation by established organizations can deter entry as well. Relentless cost reductions and quality improvement means entrants will always have to play catch-up, which does not promise substantial profits.

Mergers increase market power by changing market structure. A well-conceived, well-executed merger can reduce costs or increase market power, either of which can increase profit margins. The publicized goal of most mergers is cost reductions resulting from consolidation of some functions. The accompanying anticipation of improvement in the firm's bargaining position is usually left unspoken. Customers and suppliers usually must do business with the most powerful firms in a market. For example, failure to contract with a dominant health system will pose problems for customers and suppliers, so the system can anticipate better deals. Whether cost savings or market share gains are the more important goal of a merger is debatable.

14.5 Market Structure and Markups

Having market power does not eliminate the need to set profit-maximizing prices. Organizations should still set prices so that marginal revenue equals marginal cost (MC). If the return on equity is inadequate, the organization should exit the line of business.

14.5.1 Markups

What changes with a gain in market power is markups. A firm with substantial market power will find it profitable to set prices well above marginal cost. Figure 14.1 shows that a firm with a substantial amount of market power ($\varepsilon = -2.5$) will have a 67 percent markup. In contrast, a firm with a moderate amount of market power ($\varepsilon = -8.0$) will only have a 14 percent markup. Finally, a firm with very little market power ($\varepsilon = -12.0$) will have a 9 percent markup.

Organizations with market power benefit from markup. However, their customers face higher prices, which results in their using the product less or not at all.

As a result, managers' goals depend on whether they are buying or selling. Managers seek to reduce their suppliers' market power while increasing their own. If your suppliers have substantial market power and you have none, your profit margins will suffer.

FIGURE 14.1
Market Share
and Markups

Market Share	Market Elasticity	Firm's Elasticity	Marginal Cost	Profit-Maximizing Price
48%	−0.60	−1.25	$10.00	$50.00
24%	−0.60	−2.50	$10.00	$16.67
7.5%	−0.60	−8.00	$10.00	$11.43
5%	−0.60	−12.00	$10.00	$10.91

NOTE: This figure assumes that the firm's price elasticity equals the market elasticity divided by the firm's market share, which need not always be true.

14.5.2 The Impact of Market Structure on Markups

Analyses of the impact of market structure on markups require information on prices and costs, which is typically closely guarded by managers. There are a few healthcare studies, however, such as Nyman's (1994) on nursing homes that found higher markups in areas in which there was greater market concentration.

A market with a high degree of concentration is one with relatively few competitors or a few dominant firms. Economists often use the Hirschman-Herfindahl Index (HHI) to measure market concentration. The HHI equals the sum of the squared market shares of the competitors in a market. The HHI gets larger as the number of firms gets smaller or as the market shares of the largest firms increase. For example, a market with five firms, each of which claimed 20 percent of the market, would have an HHI of 2,000. In contrast, a market with five firms, four of which each claimed 15 percent of the market while the fifth claimed 40 percent, would have an HHI of 2,500.

The study found that a 1 percent increase in the HHI was associated with a 0.13–0.15 percent increase in prices. This might not seem like much, but it means prices would be 3 or 4 percent higher in a market with an HHI of 2,500 than in a market with an HHI of 2,000. Such a difference should have a major impact on profits.

14.6 Market Power and Profits

Market power does not guarantee profits. A firm with market power will set prices well above marginal cost but may not earn an adequate return on equity. However, firms with market power can use strategies to boost profits that firms without market power cannot.

Three competitive strategies are common among firms with market power: price discrimination, collusion, and product differentiation. We discussed price discrimination in Chapter 10; in this chapter we will focus on collusion and product differentiation.

14.6.1 Collusion

Collusion, or conspiring to limit competition, has a long history in medicine. As in other industries, the temptation to avoid the rigors of market competition can be beguiling. Collusion is profitable because demand is less elastic for the profession than for each individual participant. For example, if the price elasticity of demand for physicians' services is about −0.20 and the price elasticity of demand for an individual physician's services is about −3.00, an individual physician can increase her income by cutting prices, yet raising prices will increase the income of the profession as a whole.

Figure 14.2 shows how a 10 percent price increase would change total revenue for organizations facing different elasticities. (The change in total revenue due to price cut = [percentage change in price + percentage change in quantity] + [percentage change in price × percentage change in quantity].) For the profession as a whole, raising prices will increase revenues because demand is inelastic. For each individual professional, raising prices will reduce revenues unless other professionals change their prices, which would make demand less elastic. Of course, others are likely to respond to price cuts by cutting their own prices, so revenues will climb far less than a naive analysis would suggest.

The implication of Figure 14.2 is that physicians as a group would increase their incomes if they refused to give discounts to managed care organizations. What is good for the profession, however, is not what is good for its individual members. Individual physicians would be tempted to decry managed care discounts but make private deals with HMOs. From the perspective of the profession, penalizing defectors would prevent this problem.

FIGURE 14.2

Elasticity and Revenue Changes

Price Increase	Elasticity	Quantity Change	Revenue Change
10%	−0.1	−1%	8.9%
10%	−0.2	−2%	7.8%
10%	−0.3	−3%	6.7%
10%	−3.0	−30%	−23.0%
10%	−3.5	−35%	−28.5%
10%	−4.0	−40%	−34.0%

In the 1930s, Oregon physicians did just this. Faced with an over-supply of physicians, excess capacity in the state's hospitals, and widespread concern about the costs of healthcare, insurance companies in Oregon attempted to restrict use of physicians' services. Medical societies in Oregon responded by threatening to expel physicians who participated in these insurance plans. Because membership in a county medical society was usually a requirement for hospital privileges, this was a serious threat. This and physicians' ultimate refusal to deal with insurance companies led the insurers to abandon efforts to restrict use of physicians' services (Starr 1982).

In most industries these steps would be recognized as illegal, anti-competitive activities. However, the belief that anti-trust laws did not apply to the medical profession was widespread until a 1982 Supreme Court decision to the contrary. Since then the Federal Trade Commission has sued to prevent boycotts of insurers, efforts to deny hospital privileges to participants in managed care plans, and attempts to restrict advertising. In short, healthcare professionals and healthcare organizations are to be treated no differently than other businesses.

The benefits of collusion are clear. By restricting competition, firms can reduce the price elasticity of demand and increase markups. Collusion only increases profits, however, until it is detected.

14.7 Product Differentiation and Advertising

Product differentiation takes two forms: attribute-based and information-based. In *attribute-based* differentiation, customers recognize that two products have different attributes, even though they are fairly close substitutes, and may not respond to small price differences. In *information-based* differentiation, customers have incomplete information about how well products suit their needs. Information is expensive to gather and verify, so customers are reluctant to switch products once they have identified one that is acceptable. Both forms reduce the price elasticity of demand for a product and create market power (Caves and Williamson 1985).

Both attribute-based and information-based product differentiation are common in healthcare. For example, a board-certified pediatrician who practices on the west side of town very clearly provides a service that is different from a board-certified pediatrician who practices on the east side of town. If the two practices were closer together, more customers would view them as equivalent. Alternatively, armed only with a sense that the technical skills, interpersonal skills, and prices of surgeons can vary significantly, a potential customer who has found an acceptable surgeon is not likely to switch just because a neighbor was charged a lower fee for the same procedure. Of course, the customer might be more likely to switch if complication rates, patient satisfaction scores, and prices for both surgeons were posted on the Internet for easy comparison.

The role of information differs sharply in attribute-based and information-based product differentiation. Extensive advertising makes sense for products that differ in attributes that matter to consumers. The more clearly customers see the differences, the less elastic demand will be and the higher markups can be for "better" products. In contrast, restrictions on advertising (and even restrictions on disclosure of information) make sense when there is information-based product differentiation. The harder it is for customers to see that products do not differ in ways that matter to them, the less elastic demand will be and the higher markups can be.

The coexistence of attribute-based and information-based product differentiation in healthcare leads to confusing advertising patterns. Attribute-based product differentiation demands advertising. Getting information about product differences into the hands of customers is integral to this type of product differentiation. For example, pharmaceutical manufacturers have launched extensive direct-to-consumer advertising campaigns. On the other hand, better customer information erodes the market power created by information-based product differentiation. Where this is common, as it is in much of healthcare, there is a temptation to restrict advertising. Because private restrictions on advertising are usually illegal, the most successful limits have been based in state law.

Despite these divergent incentives, advertising has increased in recent years. One reason has been court rulings that professional societies cannot limit advertising. However, advertising has also increased in some sectors—such as inpatient care—where advertising has long been legal. The real driving force seems to be increased competition for patients.

The nature of healthcare products and the nature of healthcare markets combine to make advertising more common. Most healthcare firms have market power and competition to some degree. Advertising helps differentiate one product from another, so it increases margins. In monopoly markets (e.g., the only hospital in an isolated town), product differentiation is not useful. The provider already has high margins, and advertising is unlikely to increase them. In markets with many providers (e.g., retailers of over-the-counter pain medications), margins may be low, but it will be difficult to differentiate one seller from another and advertising expenditures will be unlikely to increase revenues.

It is difficult to assess the quality of most healthcare goods and services before using them. Because of this, advertising can perform a useful service, that of giving consumers information they would have difficulty getting otherwise. If consumers gained no information from advertising, they would probably ignore it. Having information about a product differentiates it from products about which one does not have information. Those who offer exceptional values also need to advertise to ensure that consumers are aware of their low prices or high quality. Studies of advertising in healthcare generally find that banning advertising results in higher prices.

The economic logic behind advertising and innovating is quite simple: Continue as long as the increase in revenue is greater than the increase in cost. Stop when marginal revenue from advertising or product differentiation just equals the marginal costs. This differs from the standard rule only in that the cost of differentiation (advertising or innovating) is included in the marginal costs. Figure 14.3 shows the calculations organizations need to consider. Suppose the firm starts with profits of $100,000. In case 1 it anticipates that incremental advertising costs of $10,000 will allow it to increase revenues by $50,000. Because the incremental costs of production are only $30,000, spending more on advertising makes sense in case 1. In case 2 the firm has the same production cost forecasts but anticipates that it will need to spend $22,000 on advertising to increase revenues by $50,000. The higher advertising costs in case 2 mean an attempt to increase sales would be unprofitable. As long as the incremental costs of production and advertising are less than incremental revenue, increasing advertising will increase profits. Managers need to take into account both advertising and production costs. Advertising only makes sense for products with significant margins.

The profit-maximizing amount of advertising is determined by consumers' responses to advertising and prices. The profit-maximizing rule is that advertising costs (measured as a percentage of sales) should equal $-\alpha/\varepsilon$. In other words, an organization will maximize profits when its advertising to sales ratio equals -1 times the ratio of the advertising elasticity of demand, $-\alpha$, to the price elasticity of demand, ε. The advertising elasticity of demand is the percentage increase in the quantity demanded when advertising expenses increase by 1 percent. Obviously, advertising that does not increase sales is not worth doing. Firms with less elastic

FIGURE 14.3

Advertising and Profits

	Incremental Revenue	Incremental Cost Of Production	Incremental Cost Of Advertising	Profit
Baseline				$100,000
Case 1	$50,000	$30,000	$10,000	$110,000
Case 2	$50,000	$30,000	$22,000	$98,000

Case 14.1   Deregulating Pharmaceutical Advertising

"Direct-to-consumer advertising informs and educates consumers. It lets consumers know their conditions may be treatable, and it informs consumers about the possible risks associated with pharmaceuticals. It helps them ask their doctors and pharmacists better questions. Consumers are not stupid. They understand that we are trying to sell a product and they will balance our sales pitch with information from other sources. Advertising only makes sense for products that really work. If consumers try an advertised product and it doesn't work, we have shot ourselves in the foot. Consumers won't believe our next pitch. Remember, we have $2 billion in sales, so we have a lot to lose if consumers stop trusting our brand. Advertising is information—information about products that have been rigorously reviewed for safety and effectiveness. Consumers want to know about drugs with more convenient dosing, reduced side effects, and fewer interactions. Direct-to-consumer advertising helps consumers make better choices, because, quite frankly, doctors and pharmacists are not educating the public. Deregulating direct-to-consumer advertising would be a progressive step for this country." Lee Grant stopped talking and waited for questions.

"That's a very impressive argument, Ms. Grant," said Senator Robinson. "But aren't firms using advertising to create entry barriers? And don't entry barriers result in higher prices for consumers and their insurance companies? In my view, drug companies are using advertising to differentiate their products and jack up their margins. Furthermore, this seems to be a very haphazard way of educating (and perhaps misinforming) the public. Only drugs with blockbuster potential are going to show up on television, and nobody can afford to promote a cheap, safe, and effective generic product. The drug companies are trying to get consumers to use high-priced branded products, not the inexpensive alternatives. So we wind up spending more without improving the health of the public. The case of Vioxx is instructive. It was heavily promoted, even though it had modest advantages over much less expensive products, and became a $2.5 billion blockbuster. Then we learned Vioxx increased the risks of heart attack and stroke. That was consumer education? I think we should ban direct-to-consumer advertising, not expand it."

Discussion questions:
- How could advertising be a barrier to entry?
- Could advertising reduce barriers to entry for a new product?
- Presumably drug companies are trying to differentiate their products from the competition. Will consumers be better off or worse off if the companies succeed?
- Consumers generally favor direct-to-consumer advertising, and healthcare professionals generally oppose it. Does this difference in attitudes make sense?

demand will want to spend more on advertising. A firm with an advertising elasticity of demand of 0.1 should spend 2.5 percent of its revenues on advertising if its price elasticity of demand is –4.00, but another firm with α = 0.1 should spend 5 percent of revenues on advertising if its price elasticity of demand is –2.00.

Product differentiation (through innovation or advertising) is a process, not an outcome. Differentiation, although potentially profitable, tends to erode. Product differentiation can be clear-cut (e.g., an open MRI); less distinguishable (e.g., "patient-centered care"); barely noticeable (e.g., "meals that don't taste like hospital food"); emotional (e.g., "doctors who care"); or frivolous (e.g., stripes in tooth gel). In all of these instances, however, successful differentiation asks to be copied and generally is, necessitating ceaseless efforts to differentiate products.

14.8 Conclusion

Most healthcare firms have some market power. Market power allows higher markups and can result in higher profits. As a result, firms try to acquire market power or defend the market power they have. The best way to acquire or defend market power is via regulation. Competitors find it more difficult to erode market power gained as a result of government action.

Organizations can take steps to gain market power without government action. Common strategies include preemption, limit pricing, and innovation, all of which are designed to discourage potential entrants. Mergers can also result in market power, as can collusion with rivals. Unlike other strategies for gaining market power, mergers and collusion often create legal problems. Mergers may result in public or private anti-trust lawsuits, as does collusion once it has been discovered.

Firms with market power can compete in a variety of ways. Where feasible, firms seek to gain market power via product differentiation and advertising. This makes managers' roles more challenging. Of course, the profit potential of market power creates an incentive to seek it, even without a guarantee of profits.

Homework

14.1　What does it mean to have market power? Are firms with market power extremely profitable?

14.2　Can you identify a healthcare firm with market power? What characteristics led you to choose the firm that you did?

14.3 Why would a merger reduce costs? Why would a merger increase markups? Why do many mergers fail nonetheless?

14.4 What information would you like to have to plan advertising spending?

14.5 Why might banning advertising drive up prices?

14.6 Offer examples of attribute-based product differentiation and information-based product differentiation.

14.7 Two physical therapy firms want to merge. The price elasticity of demand for physical therapy is –0.40. APT has a volume (Q) of 10,400, fixed costs (FC) of $50,000, marginal costs (MC) of $20, and a market share of 8 percent. BPT has a volume of 15,600, fixed costs of $60,000, marginal costs of $20, and a market share of 12 percent. The merged firm has a volume of 26,000, fixed costs of $100,000, marginal costs of $20, and a market share of 20 percent.
   a. What are the total costs (TC), prices, revenues, and profits for each firm and for the merged firm?
   b. How does the merger affect markups and profits?

14.8 A local hospital offered to buy APT for $5,000, and the offer was refused. However, many observers now perceive that APT is "in play" and may be sold if the right offer comes along.
   a In successful transactions, purchasers have typically paid 10 times current profits. How much would APT be worth to a buyer from outside the industry?
   b. Would you expect that BPT would be willing to pay more or less than an outside buyer?
   c. What is the most BPT would be willing to pay for APT?

14.9 Two clinics want to merge. The price elasticity of demand is –0.20, and each clinic has fixed costs of $60,000. One clinic has a volume of 7,200, marginal costs of $60, and a market share of 2 percent. The other clinic has a volume of 10,800, marginal costs of $60, and a market share of 4 percent. The merged firm would have a volume of 18,000, fixed costs of $80,000, marginal costs of $60, and a market share of 6 percent.
   a. What are the total costs, revenues, and profits for each clinic and for the merged firm?
   b. How does the merger affect markups and profits?

14.10 What would each of the clinics be worth to an outside buyer (using the guideline of 10 times annual profits)? What would each of the clinics be worth to each other?

14.11 A hospital anticipates that spending $100,000 on an advertising campaign will increase bed-days by 1,000. The marketing department anticipates that each additional bed-day will yield $2,000 in additional revenue and will increase costs by $1,200. Should the hospital proceed with the advertising campaign?

14.12 A clinic is considering reducing its advertising budget by $20,000. The clinic forecasts that visits will drop by 100 as a result. Costs are $140 per visit and revenues are $180 per visit. Should the clinic reduce its advertising budget?

14.13 The price elasticity of demand for dental services is –0.25. In a market with 100 dentists, the local dental society demanded and received an 8 percent increase in prices from the dominant dental insurance company. What should happen to the dentists' revenues and profits? (Assume that AC = MC.) Would this cartel be stable? Explain.

14.14 The marginal cost of a physician visit is $40. In a county with 50 physicians, the local medical society negotiated a rate of $90. Previously, any physician who offered discounts to an insurer or a patient could be cited for unethical behavior, be expelled from the medical society, and lose admitting privileges to the county's sole hospital. But having lost an anti-trust lawsuit, the medical society has agreed to stop enforcing its prohibitions against discounting, to allow any physician with a valid license to be a member of the medical society, and to stop linking admitting privileges to medical society membership.

   a. The price elasticity of demand for physicians' services is –0.18. What price maximizes profits for the individual physicians in the county?

   b. If all the physicians act independently, will their incomes go up or down?

   c. Is there any way the physicians could legally act to sustain a price of $90?

Chapter Glossary

Attribute-based product differentiation. Making customers aware of differences among products

Limit pricing. Setting prices low enough to discourage entry into a market

Monopolist. A firm with no rivals

Monopolistic competitor. A competitor with multiple rivals whose products are imperfect substitutes

Oligopolist. A firm with only a few rivals or a firm with only a few large rivals

Preemption. Building enough excess capacity in a market to discourage potential entrants

Price discrimination. Selling similar goods or services to different individuals at different prices

References

Bamezai, A., J. Zwanziger, G. A. Melnick, and J. M. Mann. 1999. "Price Competition and Hospital Cost Growth in the United States." *Health Economics* 8 (3): 233–43.

Capps, C., and D. Dranove. 2004. "Hospital Consolidation and Negotiated PPO Prices." *Health Affairs* 23 (2): 175–81.

Caves, R. E., and P. J. Williamson. 1985. "What Is Product Differentiation, Really?" *Journal of Industrial Economics* 34 (2): 113–32.

Dranove, D. 1998. "Economies of Scale in Non-Revenue Producing Cost Centers: Implications for Hospital Mergers." *Journal of Health Economics* 17 (1): 69–83.

Ferrier, G. D., and V. G. Valdmanis. 2004. "Do Mergers Improve Hospital Productivity?" *Journal of the Operational Research Society* 55 (10): 1071–80.

Gaynor, M., and W. B. Vogt. 2003. "Competition Among Hospitals." *Rand Journal of Economics* 34 (4): 764–85.

Keeler, E. B., G. Melnick, and J. Zwanziger. 1999. "The Changing Effects of Competition on Non-Profit and For-Profit Pricing Behavior." *Journal of Health Economics* 18 (1): 69–86.

Lee, R. H., and J. Hadley. 1981. "Physicians' Fees and Public Medical Care." *Health Services Research* 16 (2): 185–203.

McCarthy, T. R. 1985. "The Competitive Nature of the Primary-Care Physician Services Market." *Journal of Health Economics* 4 (2): 93–117.

Nyman, J. A. 1994. "The Effects of Market Concentration and Excess Demand on the Price of Nursing Home Care." *Journal of Industrial Economics* 42 (2): 193–204.

Page, S. S. 2004. "How Physicians' Organizations Compete: Protectionism and Efficiency." *Journal of Health Politics, Policy and Law* 29 (1): 75–105.

Porter, M. E. 1985. *Competitive Advantage*. New York: Free Press.

Starr, P. 1982. *The Social Transformation of American Medicine*. New York: Basic.

GOVERNMENT INTERVENTION IN HEALTHCARE MARKETS

Learning Objectives

After reading this chapter, students will be able to:

- **describe** the advantages of perfectly competitive markets,
- **explain** when markets may be inefficient, and
- **discuss** alternative approaches to market failure.

Key Concepts

- Given the right conditions, competitive markets can produce optimal outcomes.
- Markets organize vast amounts of information about costs and preferences.
- Perfectly competitive markets lead to efficient production and consumption.
- Markets are dynamically efficient.
- Most markets are imperfect.
- Markets may be inefficient when there are externalities or public goods.
- Markets may be inefficient when competition or information is imperfect.
- Efficient market outcomes may not be equitable.
- Clear assignment of property rights may improve market outcomes.
- Taxes or subsidies may improve the efficiency of some markets.
- Public provision of some products may be efficient.

15.1 Government Intervention in Healthcare

Government intervention in healthcare is extensive, even in a market-oriented society like the United States. This chapter explores the rationale for government intervention, assuming that the goal is the promotion of the public good. We will begin by looking at the virtues of markets and then examine problems with markets. The chapter concludes by considering ways that governments might intervene.

15.1.1 On the Virtues of Markets

Under the right conditions, competitive markets can lead to an allocation of resources that is *Pareto optimal*—that is, no one can be made better off without making someone worse off (Debreu 1959). These conditions are restrictive:

1. Each market should have large numbers of buyers and sellers.
2. Markets involve the sale of undifferentiated products.
3. All buyers and sellers know all of the relevant information about the market.

Markets also require maintenance of law, order, and property rights, so this list of conditions may be incomplete. Nonetheless, these conditions are seldom satisfied, leaving us with questions that are more complex and more difficult. Would relying more on markets to allocate resources make us better or worse off? Would changing the laws and regulations make us better or worse off? The difficulty is that we must choose not between perfect markets and perfect governments but between imperfect versions of each. Much of this chapter focuses on the shortcomings of markets. First, though, let's explore some of the virtues of markets.

15.1.2 Information Processing

What should the price of gasoline be? Is an additional flight between Chicago and Tulsa, Oklahoma, worth enough to consumers to justify the cost of operating it? Are consumers willing to pay for the capabilities of satellite telephones? Is there a shortage of nurses? Markets help us answer such questions.

In an ideal market, goods and services are made, distributed, and used so that the market value of production is as large as possible. The resulting prices spread information throughout the economy, coordinating the decisions of many decentralized producers and consumers. The quest for profits encourages producers to seek low-cost ways of creating the products consumers most want while using resources in the most valuable way possible. Because the decisions made by consumers are designed to maximize satisfaction, maximizing market values results in maximizing well-being. The equilibrium of an ideal market is Pareto optimal. Furthermore, market exchange is voluntary. Individuals can choose to trade or not, affording considerable freedom to participants.

In a planned economy, well-intentioned officials who use their power wisely and justly may find price setting difficult. The planning process does not automatically yield the information needed to set prices. In addition, because price setting is a political act in a planned economy, officials may have difficulty setting prices correctly even when they know the proper levels.

Case 15.1	**Setting Prices for Walkers**

Wal-Mart sells a walker called the Carex Explorer for $59.92.

Medicare covers the Explorer, but it pays over $100 (Leonhardt 2008). Since 1989, Medicare has paid for equipment such as walkers using a fee schedule equal to 95 percent of a product's average wholesale price (an unverified number provided by manufacturers). This system keeps Medicare fees substantially higher than typical retail prices (GAO 2000).

As a part of the Medicare Modernization Act of 2003, Medicare accepted bids for ten types of equipment in ten metropolitan areas. The median accepted bid was 26 percent lower than the current Medicare fee. Equipment manufacturers and retailers responded by lobbying Congress to discard the bids and delay the program, and the House of Representatives obliged by passing a bill to ditch the bids.

This example demonstrates three points. First, a well-designed bidding process can result in lower prices for public programs. Second, such programs are expensive and take a long time to set up and implement. Third, efforts to switch to a bidding process will encounter opposition from those whose profits are at risk.

Discussion questions:
- What are the risks of a bidding process like the one described in this case?
- Why would elected representatives side with the manufacturers and retailers on this issue?
- Suppose that Medicare sought bids for enough cardiac care to serve beneficiaries in your home town. What would happen economically and politically? Could you design a way of insulating Medicare from political pressure? Would you want to?
- The main problem with the current fee schedule is that Medicare overpays. What other problems might distorted fee schedules cause?

15.1.3 Static Resource Allocation

Perfectly competitive markets allocate products efficiently to the consumers most willing to pay for them. In other words, production and consumption are efficient. Products are produced as inexpensively as possible. No resources are wasted in making goods and providing services. Reorganization of production would increase costs.

Exchanges of goods and services in perfectly competitive markets all take place at the same price. As a result, consumers who value products will buy them. Products are not wasted on consumers who feel they are worth less than the amount spent to produce them.

Perfectly competitive markets result in an optimal mix of output. Their combination of least-cost production and highest-value consumption means that changes would reduce satisfaction. At the competitive optimum, price equals marginal benefit, which in turn equals marginal cost. Shifts in the output of the economy would cause the marginal cost to be higher or lower than the marginal value to consumers, which would not be optimal.

Perfectly competitive markets are not necessarily fair. Different distributions of incomes result in different market outcomes. A perfectly competitive market might lead to an efficient outcome in which most consumers have comparable incomes, or a perfectly competitive market might lead to an efficient outcome in which most consumers are ill-housed and ill-nourished and only a handful live in palaces.

15.1.4 Dynamic Resource Allocation

In a market economy, successful innovations are highly profitable. Unsuccessful innovations and inertia are highly unprofitable. As a result, markets are efficient in a dynamic sense. They respond quickly to changes in economic conditions and encourage innovation.

At the simplest level, markets squelch products that customers do not want. A product that does not create more value for potential buyers than its alternatives will fail quickly. Compounding this effect, those in authority or those with established products have difficulty preventing change; rivals are free to develop new products, and customers are free to buy them.

More important, markets reward innovation that customers want. A product that is as good as its alternatives is not likely to be more profitable than the others, whereas a better product promises high short-term profits. Customers will pay a premium for a better product, and substantial profits will follow if the market is large enough. Before too long, though, competitors will introduce similar products, and profit margins will fall. Producers must innovate continuously to maintain above-average profit margins.

Because innovation is intrinsic to market economies, we often fail to notice it. For most of human history, however, innovation was not routine. Before 1700, most people used the same technology their grandparents used. Income per capita changed little for hundreds of years (Baumol 2002).

The dynamic efficiency of markets is so important that it may trump static efficiency concerns. Suppose, for example, that a market is dominated by a few large firms. In this market, prices will be somewhat higher than they would be in a more competitive market. But, if those large firms invest more in research and development than smaller firms would, it might not be long before the resulting innovation would make consumers better off.

15.2 Market Failure

Despite their many virtues, markets do not always perform well. We will now consider the main reasons markets fail:

1. Externalities
2. Public goods
3. Imperfect competition
4. Imperfect information
5. Natural monopoly
6. Income redistribution

15.2.1 Externalities

Production or consumption of some products may directly affect others. These side effects are called *externalities*. When the side effects benefit others, they are called *external benefits*. When the side effects harm others, they are called *external costs*. When these side effects are not considered in market exchanges, the resulting equilibrium may entail volumes that are too high or too low.

For example, immunization confers external benefits on people who have not been immunized. If you are immunized, my risk of becoming ill decreases. In return for this benefit, I might be willing to pay a part of the cost of your immunization and part of the cost of others' immunizations. As a practical matter, though, I'll have a hard time providing the subsidies if there are thousands of people I want to help. I'd be able to subsidize only a small number of immunizations, which defeats the purpose of my offer.

Figure 15.1 illustrates this concept. The private demand curve, which ignores the product's external benefits, is D_P. The social demand curve, which incorporates these benefits, is D_S. The market equilibrium, which ignores the external benefits of immunization, results in a volume of Q_P. An equilibrium that takes the external benefits into account would result in the larger volume of Q_S. In short, the market equilibrium is not fully efficient.

Externalities need not be positive. If I let my untreated sewage contaminate your well, I am imposing external costs on you to have the sewage treated. I am considering the amount I would have to spend on water to get rid of wastes, but I am not considering your costs. If there were just the two of us, you could pay me to produce less sewage. If there are 100 people like me, and our sewage affects 500 or 5,000 people, these private payments will become complex and problems are likely to ensue. External benefits and costs that affect large numbers of people are characteristic of *public goods* (see section 15.2.2).

FIGURE 15.1
Market
Equilibrium
with External
Benefits

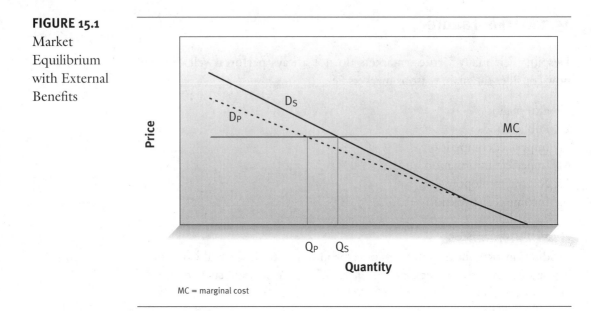

MC = marginal cost

A classic example of an externality is the *tragedy of the commons*. If everyone in a village can graze livestock on a common pasture, each person has an individual incentive to overuse the resource. The overgrazing may become so severe that all of the livestock starve and the village collapses. In other words, each person's cattle consume resources that imperil everyone else's cattle. More contemporary examples include vehicle congestion in cities, in which each driver ignores the costs imposed on others; overuse of the Ogallala aquifer in the central United States, in which each farmer's pumping increases costs for others; and excessive production of greenhouse gases by one country that causes a climate change affecting all countries.

The use of antibiotics in healthcare is another example of the tragedy of the commons. Patients benefit from the liberal use of antibiotics, but society suffers because overuse speeds the development of antibiotic-resistant strains.

The flip side of the tragedy of the commons is a *network externality*—a value each additional user adds for existing users. Communications equipment of all sorts promotes network externalities. Electronic health record systems are a good example. An electronic health record system is valuable to a hospital. It transmits records quickly throughout the hospital, and any physician can instantly access a patient's record. If the other hospitals in town adopt compatible systems, the value of that electronic health record system increases. Its value increases further if all providers in the country adopt compatible systems. The hospital will be able to offer more appropriate treatment to an emergency department patient from another town because it will have access to that patient's past treatments, test results, and vital signs.

Standards also promote network externalities. For example, one reason why healthcare costs are high in the United States is the absence of widely accepted standards for billing. Insurers have their own systems, and providers must submit bills in a wide range of formats to be paid in a timely fashion. If two insurers adopt a common standard, they will save some money, but hospitals and clinics (which are not parties to the decision to standardize) will save even more. The value of this standardization increases as more and more insurers join.

15.2.2 Public Goods

A public good is an extreme example of externalities. A pure public good has two unusual characteristics: Consumption by one person does not prevent consumption by another, and exclusion is difficult. One person's use of a pure public good does not interfere with another's use of it, so use is *nonrival*: The marginal cost of letting one more person use the public good is zero. For instance, my enjoyment of clean air in the country does not limit your enjoyment of it. Alternatively, I can use the new research you are using. In addition, preventing people from using pure public goods is difficult, so consumption is *nonexcludable*, meaning that everyone has access to them.

A radio broadcast illustrates the difference between these two concepts. When a program is broadcast, anyone in the reception area can get the signal. Adding another listener does not affect current listeners, so consumption of the broadcast is clearly nonrival. In contrast, a radio broadcast may or may not be excludable. Most commercial radio in the United States does not exclude any potential listeners, but Sirius Satellite Radio is only available to subscribers, so exclusion is possible. Because exclusion is possible, radio broadcasts are not public goods.

In contrast, a reduction in levels of sulphur dioxide in the air is a public good. One person's enjoyment of better air quality does not prevent another person from enjoying it too, so consumption of improved air quality is nonrival. In addition, it is hard to imagine that anyone could be prevented from taking advantage of cleaner air, so consumption is nonexcludable.

Markets are not likely to result in the right amounts of public goods being consumed. If market transactions lead to any consumption of public goods, the quantities are likely to be too small.

Because everyone can simultaneously enjoy a public good, the marginal benefit of a public good equals the sum of the marginal benefits for everyone in society. So, if a 1 percent reduction in sulphur dioxide (SO_2) in the atmosphere is worth $1 to Jordan, $2 to Kim, and $4 to Logan, it will be worth $7 to the three of them. The marginal benefit to society is the sum of the marginal benefits to the members of society, and the members of our

---

Case 15.2   **To Vaccinate or Not**

"Look, the chicken pox vaccine comes with some risks. The chicken pox vaccine is a live attenuated vaccine. It can cause a mild case of chicken pox or shingles. Plus, it's not necessary. As long as everyone else at work has had chicken pox or has been vaccinated, I don't need to be vaccinated. Plus, I don't like needles or doctors."

"But Cameron," replied Kim, "what if everyone or a third of the population followed your example? Then there would be no herd immunity. Everyone who had not been vaccinated would be at risk. In addition, chicken pox is a different disease in adults. The rash is usually more widespread, the fever lasts longer, and complications are more common. And if a pregnant woman gets chicken pox, a lot of really nasty things can happen to her baby. I know it takes two shots, I know you don't want to spend the money, and I know you hate shots. But you really ought to get vaccinated, for yourself and for the other people here at work."

Discussion questions:
- What are the external effects of a vaccine?
- Would too few people be vaccinated if it were not mandatory? What evidence supports your conclusion?
- What steps do governments take to increase vaccination rates?
- What steps do private companies take to increase vaccination rates? Why?

---

three-person society should be seeking an outcome in which the marginal benefit to society equals the marginal cost.

Figure 15.2 illustrates this situation. If the three members of society act independently, only Logan will pay for sulphur dioxide reduction and the level chosen will be 1 percent. In this example Logan's marginal benefit equals $4.25 minus 25 times the reduction in sulphur dioxide, which amounts to $4 for a 1 percent reduction. (A marginal benefit schedule like this is simply a recasting of a demand curve in terms of value at each level of consumption.) The marginal cost is $3.60 plus 40 times the reduction in sulphur dioxide, so the marginal cost also equals $4 for a 1 percent reduction.

At this cost Jordan and Kim will be unwilling to pay for any reduction in sulphur dioxide, although they will benefit from Logan's spending. In this example Jordan's marginal benefit schedule is 1.4 minus 40 times the extent of sulphur dioxide reduction, and Kim's marginal benefit schedule is 2.24 minus 25 times the extent of sulphur dioxide reduction. So, Jordan would only be willing to spend $1 for a 1 percent reduction and Kim would be willing to pay $2. However, they will be willing to pay for a much larger

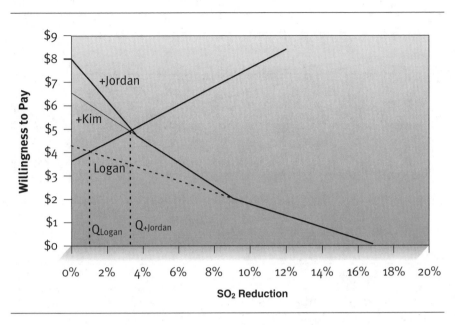

FIGURE 15.2
Demand for a
Public Good

reduction in sulphur dioxide if they recognize that reducing sulphur dioxide levels is a public good and pool their resources. In this example they will be willing to pay for a 3.306 percent reduction in sulphur dioxide, with Logan paying $3.42, Kim paying $1.42, and Jordan paying $0.08. The sum of these marginal benefits is $4.92, which is equal to the marginal cost. This level of reduction, which equates the marginal benefit and marginal cost, would be optimal for this three-person society.

So, cooperation could lead to an optimal result. The difficulty is that Jordan would be even better off if Kim and Logan paid for the reduction in sulphur dioxide. After all, Jordan will benefit whether he pays or not. This is called the *free rider* problem. In a three-person society everyone could probably be persuaded to pay, but it is less clear that this will be true if there are 3 million or 300 million people in a society.

15.2.3 Imperfect Competition

At equilibrium in a perfectly competitive market, price equals marginal cost. Producing more volume than that produced at equilibrium would be inefficient because the value of the additional output would be less than its cost. In an imperfectly competitive market, however, every producer has some market power, so producers will set prices to make marginal revenue equal marginal cost.

Figure 15.3 illustrates an imperfectly competitive market. Marginal cost (MC) is $60. To maximize profits, the producer sets a price of $80, which yields marginal revenue (MR) of $60. As a result, some customers who would be willing to pay more than marginal cost, but not $80, would

FIGURE 15.3
Imperfect
Markets and
Market
Outcomes

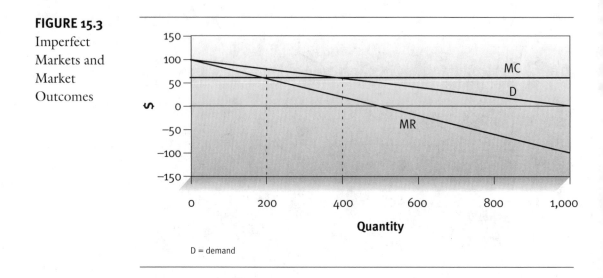

D = demand

not buy this product. In a perfectly competitive market, the price would be $60 and volume would be twice as large.

15.2.4 Imperfect Information and Incomplete Markets

The efficiency of market outcomes rests on the assumption that buyers and sellers have perfect information, which is seldom the case in healthcare. As Arrow (1963) argued, the purpose of a visit to a physician is often the reduction of uncertainty; people seek care because they need more complete information. If patients are unsure about the benefit they will gain from a physician visit, they may decide to forgo the visit, which can lead to less-than-optimal market outcomes.

Figure 15.4 illustrates three possible outcomes for the scenario above. D_1, D_2, and D_3 describe different consumers' willingness to pay for care. D_1 represents the willingness of a consumer who correctly understands the value of a physician visit. Given the marginal cost of producing this information, the consumer will buy Q_1. D_2 describes the willingness of a consumer who overstates the value of a physician visit. She will buy Q_2, which is substantially larger than Q_1. More important, the true value of the visit at Q_2 is well below marginal cost. (The true value lies on the D_1 demand curve.) This consumer would be better off if she reallocated spending to other products. Finally, D_3 describes the willingness of a consumer who understates the value of a physician visit. In this example, he makes no visits and forgoes all the benefits those visits might have provided. He would be better off if he reallocated spending from other areas to physician visits. In short, we cannot be sure that the market outcome will be optimal if information is imperfect.

The situation is even more complex than Figure 15.4 suggests. Physicians and other experts may have discretion in recommending services. Even after a service has been provided, the consumer may have difficulty

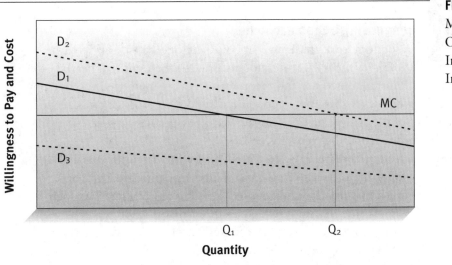

FIGURE 15.4
Market
Outcomes with
Imperfect
Information

ascertaining whether the expert made the best recommendation, especially if the expert reaps large profits from the recommended service. Insurance further complicates matters. Insurers have difficulty tracking the true costs of services, and the conventional wisdom is that slow adjustments in insurance fees distort the profitability of some services. For example, the cost of MRI equipment has dropped sharply even as the quality of images has increased and the time needed to obtain an image has gone down. As a result, the cost of producing a scan has dropped, but prices for scans have come down only slowly. As a result, MRI scans have become so profitable that many individual physicians have begun installing them in their offices and use of MRI scans has exploded (Abelson 2004).

15.2.5 Natural Monopoly

If fixed costs are so high that only one firm can survive in the long run, that firm is a *natural monopoly*. Monopolies develop relative to the structure of costs and the size of the market. In a small market, only one hospital may be able to survive. In a larger market, multiple competitors can thrive.

The larger the investment needed to set up a firm, the more likely the firm will be a natural monopoly. If an imaging center has fixed costs of $20 million, it will be a natural monopoly in many markets. If an imaging center has fixed costs of $2 million, it will be a natural monopoly only in the smallest markets. Like any monopoly, natural monopolies tend to sell their products and services at overly high prices, resulting in low sales.

15.2.6 Income Redistribution

A substantial part of government spending can be described as insurance or redistribution. Medicaid and Social Security Disability Insurance are examples.

Case 15.3	**Diagnosing a Stomach Ache**

A sophomore at the University of Richmond had a stomach ache (CBS News 2007). It did not go away, so she went to a nearby emergency room. Physicians examined her and recommended a computerized tomography (CT) scan. A CT scan uses X-rays and computer technology to produce cross-sectional images of any part of the body. The CT scan showed a benign ovarian cyst. No treatment was recommended, and the pain subsided.

Shortly thereafter, her father received a bill for $8,500 from the hospital, $6,500 of which was for the CT scan. A physician himself, he protested that his daughter's symptoms should have been diagnosed from her medical history, a pelvic examination, and perhaps an ultrasound (which costs less than $1,500).

The hospital argued that his diagnostic strategy would not have ruled out appendicitis or kidney stones. Agreeing, her father pointed out that a CT scan could always be done if a patient's history, examination, and ultrasound failed to produce a clear diagnosis.

To make matters worse, other hospitals were charging less than $1,200 for abdominal CT scans. Medicare and most insurance plans pay less than $1,200.

Discussion questions:
- After reading this case, would you be more or less willing to have a CT scan done if an emergency room physician recommended it? How confident would you be that your choice was a good one?
- Had she asked her physicians what the alternatives were, they probably would have discussed watchful waiting and immediate ultrasound. Would you expect a college student to ask for alternatives? Explain your logic.
- How can consumers make a good choice without information about price? Emergency department staff are unlikely to know the list prices or allowed fees for a CT scan.
- Do you think hospitals should be required to provide an estimate of the cost of elective procedures before a patient chooses to have one done? Explain your logic.
- Do you think information about prices would have influenced the patient's decision or the physicians' recommendations?

Taxes are levied on the healthy and wealthy to provide medical care and income to those less fortunate.

Redistribution is usually rationalized in one of two ways. One views redistribution as a public good. We all have some sympathy for the unfortunate, and we all benefit if someone offers them aid. Individual gains are small, however, and we may be tempted to let others provide our share of the redistribution. People who obtain a benefit at another's expense or without the usual cost or effort are called *free riders*. Free riding results in underprovision of the public good.

A related approach introduced by John Rawls (1971) argues that if we were ignorant of our circumstances, we would want a society that allowed for some redistribution. In this approach, we would decide on how much redistribution was appropriate behind a "veil of ignorance," meaning we would not know whether we were healthy or unhealthy, wealthy or poor.

15.3 Remedies

The remainder of this chapter explores possible remedies for market failure. Remember that doing nothing is always an option. Government intervention will not necessarily improve the situation. Governments also fail, and intervention could even worsen the situation.

15.3.1 Assignment of Property Rights

Many externalities result from ambiguities about the ownership of property rights. For example, does a downstream city have a right to clean water, or does an upstream city have a right to use a river as a sewer? Often the first step in solving externality problems is defining who has the right to use an asset. Once users are defined, asset sales, private agreements, regulations, or taxes can be used to produce efficient outcomes.

An influential analysis by Coase (1960) pointed out that ambiguity about property rights underlies many externality problems. As long as the costs of reaching and enforcing an agreement are small, the people involved in an externality case can reach agreements that solve the problem. For example, if the upstream city has the right to pollute, the downstream city can pay it to refrain from polluting the river. If the downstream city has the right to pure water, the upstream city will have to pay for the right to pollute (and will usually find it can pay less if it limits its pollution). Either way, the property owners can reach an efficient solution. With unclear property rights, who should pay whom is unclear, and too much of the externality is likely to be produced. If it is not clear that the upstream city has to pay for the right to pollute or it is not clear that the downstream city has to pay to prevent pollution, the upstream city is likely to underestimate the cost of pollution as a way of disposing of waste and dump too much waste into the water.

If an externality affects many people or is caused by many people, the costs of reaching and enforcing an agreement will be high. As a result, workable private agreements will be hard to reach. For example, pollution of Chesapeake Bay is caused by millions of people and affects millions of people. In such cases, governments typically claim property rights and use a variety of tools to improve outcomes.

In recent years, governments have taken steps to create markets for pollutants. First, the government asserts its ownership of the property right affected by pollution. Then, firms or jurisdictions are issued permits to pollute. These permits are worth more to firms or jurisdictions that have difficulty reducing pollution and are worth less to firms that reduce pollution more easily. Trades among potential polluters establish a price per unit of pollution and push potential polluters to equalize the costs of pollution reduction. Firms that incur low costs to reduce pollution have an incentive to do more to clean up than do firms that incur high costs to reduce pollution; the latter buy permits so they can limit their cleanup efforts.

The 1990 Clean Air Act amendments set national caps for emission of sulfur dioxide by power plants, issued permits equal to this cap to plants, and allowed plants to trade permits. This program significantly reduced emissions of sulfur dioxide, and most observers consider it a success. The price of compliance was low, so compliance was high, and firms were encouraged to innovate to reduce emissions.

15.3.2 Taxes and Subsidies

If a product generates significant external benefits, a subsidy can be used to make the market outcome more efficient. Whether the subsidy goes to producers or consumers does not matter. Either way, the market price will fall and consumption will rise.

Figure 15.5 illustrates the effects of a subsidy. The demand curve D_1 describes the willingness of consumers to pay for a product. Because it yields external benefits, the market outcome will be Q_1, which is inefficiently small. Giving consumers a subsidy (S) will expand consumption to Q_2, which will be the efficient level if the right subsidy has been chosen. Alternatively, one could subsidize producers, thereby reducing the marginal cost by S. This subsidy will also cause consumption to increase to Q_2.

If this product generated external costs, a tax could be imposed to reduce consumption. The challenge with the tax or subsidy is determining the appropriate rate. Changing tax or subsidy rates is not an easy political process, and the market will not always make the appropriate rate evident.

15.3.3 Public Production

Public provision of products is another approach to market failure. Public provision is especially useful for pure public goods. When there are significant externalities and excluding certain potential customers is difficult or inefficient, public provision may be the best response. Even if private firms can profitably produce some of the output consumers seek, using prices (as private firms must) to pay for such products is undesirable. For example, private

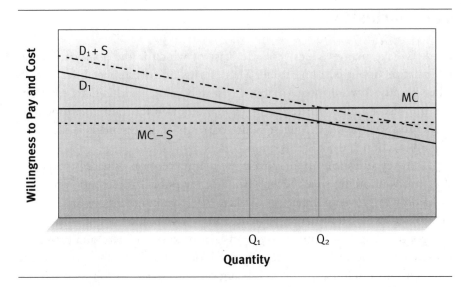

FIGURE 15.5
Market
Outcomes with
a Subsidy

research firms might be able to profitably conduct some public health research by disseminating the results only to organizations that pay to get access to it. But this is inefficient, because too few people will get access to the research. The cost of sharing the results with additional organizations is very small, and the value of the research is not reduced if it is more widely shared.

If redistribution is a goal, using prices to affect product consumption may also be undesirable. For example, prices that are high enough to allow a clinic to survive may also be high enough to prevent low-income citizens from using the clinic.

Public provision does not necessarily mean public production. For example, medical research has many of the attributes of public goods. Although government employees perform medical research, a large share of research is performed by scholars who are not government employees, but private researchers competing for tax-supported research funds. In another example of public provision with private production, medical care for the poor is usually provided to improve the health of our least fortunate citizens, meaning that the goal is largely redistribution. In some cases, this care is provided by government hospitals and clinics. More commonly, though, care is provided by private hospitals and clinics but funded by tax-supported programs like Medicaid.

15.3.4 Regulation
The next chapter examines regulation. Regulation is an important form of government intervention in markets, especially in healthcare. Markets need rules to work, so regulation is not an alternative to markets. Some regulations cause markets to work well; other regulations have the opposite effect.

15.4 Conclusion

Markets have many virtues, not the least of which is the ability to reveal information about cost and value. Many forms of government intervention falter because key information about cost and value is lacking. In addition, the impulse to innovate inherent in markets is important for improved health and well-being. A long-standing criticism of governments is their bias toward inaction and the status quo.

A key question about government intervention is hard to answer: Will intervention improve the well-being of the public? Intervention will not necessarily improve an imperfect market. Effective interventions are hard to design and even harder to implement. In the rough-and-tumble of political life, good intentions do not always translate into good effects, and proposals backed by advocates are not always good ideas. Furthermore, government interventions can improve the well-being of individuals or groups even if the interventions do not improve overall well-being.

This critique should not be pushed too far. There are problems with government support for research, but there seems to be a strong consensus that the overall benefits are considerable and that government action is necessary. There are problems with the government's public health activities, but there is no consensus that ending these activities would make our citizens better off. On the other hand, some interventions should be ended. The challenge is to determine what new programs to start and which existing programs to expand, contract, or terminate.

Homework

15.1   Global warming is a classic example of a public good. Analyze this comment and explain your answer.

15.2   The existence of market failure does not signal what should be done in response. Analyze this comment and explain your answer.

15.3   Imperfect competition is the norm, so healthcare markets cannot work. Analyze this comment and explain your answer.

15.4   Markets work; governments do not. Analyze this comment and explain your answer.

15.5   Are market forces strong enough to deliver efficient healthcare?

15.6   For each scenario, assess whether there is an externality.

   a.   Vaccinating children against influenza reduces its incidence among the elderly.

   b.   Newly graduated nurses flock to teaching hospitals for training. After working for a year, many leave to work for competitors.

    c. A couple who planned to move to Florida to retire find that the plummeting housing market has wiped out their equity.

    d. A physician complains that she spends a third of her time explaining to patients why television advertisements about medications for their conditions do not apply to them.

15.7 The supply of measles vaccine is given by $Q = 450 \times P$. The demand for measles vaccine is given by $Q = 20,000 - 50 \times P$.

    a. What is the market equilibrium price and quantity?

    b. The demand curve implies that private willingness to pay is $P = 400 - Q/50$. However, there are external benefits associated with each measles vaccination, so the social demand curve is $Q = 20,000 - 50 \times (P - 5)$. What are the equilibrium price and quantity if these external benefits are considered?

    c. Propose an intervention that will result in this equilibrium volume.

15.8 The supply of an antibiotic is $Q = 30 \times P - 200$. The demand for it is $Q = 8,800 - 20 \times P$.

    a. What is the market equilibrium price and quantity?

    b. Use of the antibiotic creates $20 in external costs due to water pollution. Would the market outcome be different if a $20 tax were levied on producers instead?

15.9 Vaccination schedules are predictable, meaning insurance coverage for vaccinations does not protect consumers against risks. Insurance coverage for vaccinations drives up costs because more people get vaccinated if coverage is available and because insurers have overhead costs. Does insurance coverage for vaccines do anything useful? Explain your answer.

15.10 About two-thirds of funding for substance abuse treatment comes from taxpayers. Are there external benefits of substance abuse treatment that warrant this level of public funding?

15.11 Provide examples of the following types of government intervention in healthcare:

    a. Government production

    b. Subsidies for products

    c. Taxes on products

    d. Price regulation

    e. Quality regulation

    f. Inaction

15.12 Provide healthcare examples of the following types of market failure:

    a. External benefits

    b. External costs

    c. Public goods

    d. Imperfect competition

    e. Imperfect information

15.13 Private foundations support medical research. Doesn't their support make tax funding of medical research unnecessary?

15.14 Public health information can be broadcast at a cost of $100. Public health information is a pure public good, in that many people can use the information simultaneously and in that preventing people from using the information is very difficult. One group of residents has a demand curve for public health information of the form $Q = 50 - P$. Here Q is the number of public health broadcasts per month and P is the price per broadcast. Another group has a demand curve of $Q = 140 - P$.

    a. At a price of $100 per broadcast, how many broadcasts per month will be demanded? (Add the quantities demanded by each group.)

    b. What is the total willingness to pay for 85 broadcasts? (Recast the demand curve to reveal willingness to pay and add the amounts for the two groups. For one group willingness to pay equals $50 - Q$. For the other it equals $140 - Q$. For both groups the minimum is $0.)

    c. At what level of output does willingness to pay equal $100?

    d. What do these results imply?

15.15 Every 1 percent reduction in the level of particulates in the air costs $200,000. Low-income residents in a region have a demand for particulate reduction of $R = 10 - P$ (R is the level of particulate reduction and P is the price per 1 percent reduction). High-income residents have a demand for particulate reduction of $R = 40 - 2P$.

    a. Is reduction of the level of particulates a public or private good?

    b. What will the market demand for particulate reduction be?

    c. What is the optimal level of particulate reduction?

15.16 Few orthopedic surgeons publish data describing their surgical volumes, infection rates, mortality rates, functional gain rates, or customer satisfaction rates.

    a. How much would a regulation requiring publication of such data cost?

    b. Would such a regulation improve the workings of the market?

    c. Would such regulation be an appropriate government activity?

    d. Do we need a regulation requiring publication of data for surgeons if private physician rating firms already exist?

Chapter Glossary

External benefit. A positive impact of a transaction for a consumer or producer not involved in the transaction

External cost. A negative impact of a transaction for a consumer or producer not involved in the transaction

Externality. A benefit or cost imposed on someone who is not a party to the transaction that causes it

Free rider. Someone who benefits from a public good without bearing its cost

Network externality. The effect each additional user of a product or service has on the value of that product or service to existing users

Nonrival consumption. Consumption by one person that does not prevent simultaneous consumption by another person

Nonexcludable consumption. Nonpreventable consumption by someone who did not pay for a good or service

Pareto optimal. An allocation of resources is Pareto optimal if no reallocation of resources is possible that will improve the well-being of one person without worsening the well-being of another.

Public good. A good whose consumption is nonrival and nonexcludable

Tragedy of the commons. Over- or underuse of a resource that occurs when ownership of the resource is unclear and users produce externalities

References

Abelson, R. 2004. "An M.R.I. Machine for Every Doctor? Someone Has to Pay." [Online article; retrieved 1/23/09.] http://query.nytimes.com/gst/fullpage.html?res=9C04E0D7113EF930A25750C0A9629C8B63&sec=&spon=&&scp=1&sq=abelson%20mri&st=cse.

Arrow, K. J. 1963. "Uncertainty and the Welfare Economics of Medical Care." *American Economic Review* 53 (5): 941–73.

Baumol, W. J. 2002. *The Free-Market Innovation Machine: Analyzing the Growth Miracle of Capital.* Princeton, NJ: Princeton University Press.

CBS News. 2007. "Defensive Medicine: Cautious or Costly?" [Online information; retrieved 7/2/08.] www.cbsnews.com/stories/2007/10/22/eveningnews/main3394654.shtml.

Coase, R. 1960. "The Problem of Social Cost." *Journal of Law and Economics* 3: 1–44.

Debreu, G. 1959. *Theory of Value*. New York: Wiley.

Government Accountability Office (GAO). 2000. "Use of Revised 'Inherent Reasonableness' Process Generally Appropriate." [Online information; retrieved 6/28/08.] www.gao.gov/archive/2000/he00079.pdf.

Leonhardt, D. 2008. "High Medicare Costs, Courtesy of Congress." [Online information; retrieved 6/28/08.] www.nytimes.com/2008/06/25/business/25leonhardt.html.

Rawls, J. 1971. *A Theory of Justice*. Cambridge, MA: Harvard University Press.

REGULATION

After reading this chapter, students will be able to:

- **describe** the importance of regulation for managers;
- **explain** the interest group model of regulation;
- **analyze** the effects of regulations on firms, rivals, and consumers; and
- **discuss** alternative approaches to market failure.

- Healthcare is extensively regulated.
- Regulation can make or break an organization (or its competitors).
- The objective of regulation is consumer protection.
- The rationale for consumer protection regulations is consumer ignorance.
- Legislation and regulation reflect interest group politics.
- When markets are imperfect, regulation cannot always improve outcomes.
- Providers are likely to "capture" the regulatory process.
- Market responses to consumer ignorance can limit the need for regulation.

16.1 Introduction

Healthcare is extensively regulated, and new regulations are constantly under consideration. Regulation is important to managers for five reasons:

1. Changes to regulations can make or break an organization. For example, in 1998 the federal government required that home healthcare firms obtain surety bonds to participate in Medicare. This regulation was later rescinded, but by that time it had already caused many firms to go out of business.

2. In some circumstances, firms can use regulations to gain a competitive edge, especially when the regulations can be used to prevent entry by a potential rival. For example, Armstrong Memorial Hospital was able to use the Pennsylvania certificate of need law to prevent the construction of a competing ambulatory surgery center (U.S. Department of Justice 2000). Claims of regulatory violations by competitors can delay or derail projects, even if the claims are ultimately dismissed. For these reasons, managers must understand the impact of regulations on their organizations, react effectively to changes to regulations, and know when political action is necessary.

3. Managers need to understand the impetus behind healthcare regulation. Regulations are politically acceptable because the complexity of healthcare makes consumers feel vulnerable. Healthcare organizations must address these feelings of vulnerability, as failure to do so invites additional regulation or loss of business.

4. Managers need to understand that legislating and regulating are continuing political contests. Most organizations have little to gain and much to lose in these risky contests. Few organizations can command enough political power to win lasting advantages through the political process, but all organizations need to be aware of the threats these contests pose.

5. Some regulations work poorly because they conflict with powerful financial incentives. Many of the same incentives that reinforce or undermine regulations also affect private contracts. Managers must know when regulations or contracts will work and when incentives will undermine them.

As noted in Chapter 15, markets and regulation are inseparable. Markets function badly with poorly designed rules, and regulations work badly when they conflict with market incentives. How well a healthcare market functions depends crucially on its regulatory structure.

16.2 Market Imperfections

Objections to regulation often stress that unfettered markets serve consumers well. This assertion may be true for perfectly competitive markets, but most healthcare markets fall far short of this ideal. At the heart of these imperfections lies "rational consumer ignorance," or consumers' inability to make good choices. Before we discuss this important issue in healthcare regulation, let's look at the three other main imperfections that beset healthcare markets: insurance, market power, and externalities.

16.2.1 Insurance

By distorting consumers' incentives, insurance reduces the likelihood that healthcare markets will function ideally. Patients are shielded from the true costs of healthcare, and even the most ethical provider will feel comfortable recommending goods and services that the patient would be unwilling to buy if he or she faced the full cost. Moreover, the healthcare system in the United States limits the role of consumers in choosing insurance plans. Because patients are insulated from the true costs of care, their healthcare choices are unlikely to fully reflect their values. This lack of connection between what consumers value and what healthcare products cost is an important market imperfection.

16.2.2 Market Power

Most healthcare providers have some market power, which means prices will exceed marginal cost. To guarantee that markets will allocate resources at least as well as any other system, prices need to reflect the opportunity cost of using a good or service. By driving a wedge between the costs and prices of products, market power compounds the distortions introduced by insurance and may cause markets to function poorly. Moreover, in markets with firms that have market power, price controls can be useful tools. In a perfectly competitive market, price controls can be irrelevant (when market prices fall below regulated levels) or harmful (when market prices rise above regulated levels). When organizations have significant market power, a third outcome is possible: Price controls can result in lower prices and higher output. Price controls are not guaranteed to work in such markets, however; they can still be irrelevant or harmful. But price controls can be beneficial if the distortions they create are smaller than the distortions they remove.

16.2.3 Externalities

Some healthcare issues involve significant externalities. As we noted in Chapter 15, an *externality* is a benefit received by, or a cost imposed on, someone who is not a party to a transaction. For example, installation of a catalytic converter in a car in Los Angeles will make the air cleaner not only for the owner of the car but also for others who live there and across the country. Markets tend not to work well when externalities are significant. Consumers and producers generally focus on the private benefits of transactions, which results in underconsumption of products that generate external benefits and overconsumption of products that generate external costs. Not surprisingly, the regulatory role of government tends to be substantial in these instances. For example, consider three activities that generate externalities: the search for new knowledge, the control of communicable diseases, and the maintenance of the environment. Patent and copyright laws restrict use of new knowledge, so producers are able to profit from selling it and thus are motivated to produce it. Public health regulations can mandate immunizations or require treatment of those infected with communicable diseases. Environmental regulations may restrict how resources are used or effectively change ownership rights. The details of these regulations can be controversial, but few societies leave resource allocation in such areas entirely to market forces.

16.3 Rational Consumer Ignorance

Healthcare regulations serve multiple purposes, but the ostensible objective of most regulations has long been consumer protection. The argument is that consumers need protection because they are rationally ignorant about the healthcare choices they must make.

At some point, everyone has difficulty making healthcare choices. In many cases decision makers have to rely on ambiguous or incomplete information. Although the scientific aura of modern medicine may suggest otherwise, many therapies lack a firm scientific basis. Even when the scientific evidence is good (in cases where investigators have carried out controlled clinical trials), decision makers may have a hard time applying it. Moreover, the results of controlled trials do not always translate to the uncontrolled environment of community practice. Even valid evidence involves probabilities, and most of us (including most healthcare providers) have difficulty using this sort of information well. We tend to see patterns where there are none, place too much emphasis on cases that are memorable or recent, and ignore the rules of probability.

Patients face additional problems. They often must make decisions when they do not feel well and are experiencing a great deal of stress. They typically lack the experience, information, and skills they need to make healthcare choices. Even after they have chosen a course of action, consumers may have difficulty assessing whether they were diagnosed correctly, whether they were prescribed the right therapy, and whether that therapy was executed properly.

The ignorance of most patients is explainable. Few of us know the healthcare choices we will have to make or when we will have to make them. We don't want to invest the time to inform ourselves because we might not ever use the information. We'd rather have somebody else do the research. Of course, rational ignorance is not universal. Patients with chronic illnesses often are well informed about their care because they expect to make ongoing decisions and are motivated to become knowledgeable.

Consumers' struggle with medical decisions makes them vulnerable in a number of ways. Consumers often do not know when to seek care. They can have difficulty evaluating the recommendations of healthcare professionals, the quality of care, or the price of that care. They may be unable to differentiate care that is worth more from care that costs more. To reduce their vulnerability, consumers may turn to medical professionals for advice.

Unfortunately, securing provider recommendations does not render consumers unassailable. Providers often have incentives to be imperfect agents. A provider may sell a product because he or she is being paid by the producer to sell it, or may recommend a therapy because it is more profitable than another treatment. Patients may wind up undergoing treatment that is ineffective or harmful, or taking the advice of incompetent or unethical providers. In short, relying on providers for advice can reduce, but not necessarily efface, consumers' vulnerability.

For these reasons, providers have an interest in reducing consumers' concerns about their vulnerability. Consumers who cannot distinguish good advice from bad may ignore all of it. Consumers who cannot distinguish reliable from unreliable healthcare professionals may decide to forgo care. Regulations serve provider interests by signaling quality to consumers. As long as competent, trustworthy professionals find it easier to live with the regulations than incompetent, untrustworthy professionals do, regulations can be useful for both consumers and providers. Indeed, this is one reason much of the demand for regulation comes from the groups to be regulated and why there is so much self-regulation. For example, a group of physicians with a particular specialty may decide to create its own regulations that it expects will keep lesser-qualified physicians out of the specialty. This would help the group's own market share, and help the public.

Rational ignorance and distortions induced by insurance, market power, and externalities will continue to make healthcare markets imperfect. Remember, however, that market regulation of such influences does not guarantee improved outcomes. Regulations are usually imperfectly designed and imperfectly implemented. In addition, regulations' consumer protection rationale may be just that: a rationale. Regulations can be used to gain a competitive advantage and may harm, not help, consumers.

16.4 The Interest Group Model of Regulation

Legislation need not serve the public interest. Noting that groups can use regulations to expand their markets and gain market power, the *interest group model of regulation* argues that legislatures are similar to markets, in that individuals and groups seek regulations to further their interests. Regulatory barriers to competition are often better than other competitive advantages because they are often harder for competitors to breach (especially for new firms or firms from outside an area, which have little or no political influence). Product features can be duplicated and marketing plans can be copied by even the most insignificant startup firm, but large, well-established firms have significant political advantage.

16.4.1 Limiting Competition

One of the best ways to gain market power is to limit competition. Regulation is an effective way of doing this. For example, when confronted by the development of freestanding ambulatory surgical centers, the American Hospital Association sought to use state certificate of need laws to restrict their expansion. Similarly, dental societies have long supported state laws prohibiting persons not licensed as dentists to fit and dispense dentures. Although lobbying the legislature to pass laws to prevent competition is legal, working together to prevent competition is illegal. In addition, the industry being regulated is likely to control the regulatory process, so consumer protection legislation may represent "existing firm protection" and not the consumer. Managers cannot ignore politics; doing so can put an organization at risk.

16.4.2 Licensure

Licensure is professional control of the regulatory process. A profession can be regulated in many ways. Professional regulation often protects the economic interests of the regulated group far better than it protects the health and safety interests of the public. States generally regulate health professionals via licensure, certification, and registration. Licensure prohibits people from performing the duties of a profession without meeting requirements set by the state. Certification prohibits those who do not meet requirements set by the state from using a title, but not from practicing. Registration requires practitioners to file their names, addresses, and relevant qualifications.

Licensure is the most restrictive form of regulation. It can prohibit practice by individuals without the right qualifications or require that they practice under the supervision of another professional. Its use is often justified by concerns about safety. While recognizing that certification considerably reduces consumer ignorance, advocates of licensure contend that it prevents unwary consumers from making unsafe choices. In some cases, however, licensure can prevent consumers from making choices that might make sense for them. Furthermore, it forces consumers to use highly trained, expensive personnel when there may be viable alternatives.

16.4.3 Regulation as a Competitive Strategy

Regulations that affect the structure or process of an organization's operations typically increase its costs and reduce its flexibility. Naturally, firms resist regulation (even if their business plans are consistent with the goals of the regulation). For these reasons, imposing regulations on rivals (but not

Case 16.1	**Lay Midwifery**

"We license nurse midwives for a good reason—to protect the safety of our citizens. Medicine should be practiced only by licensed professionals. Lay midwives enter the profession via independent midwifery school or apprenticeship and have substantially less training than a physician or a professional nurse midwife. Thirty-six states restrict or prohibit the practice of lay midwifery, and many hospitals will not grant privileges to professionals who assist in home deliveries. No credible case can be made for allowing the practice of lay midwifery. The American College of Obstetricians and Gynecologists does not support the provision of care by lay midwives," testified Leslie.

"Opponents of lay midwifery usually cite safety concerns, but the evidence does not support their case," argued Kelly. "Johnson and Daviss (2005), who have no axe to grind, show that the outcomes of home births assisted by certified professional midwives are comparable to those of low-risk hospital births. The quality argument is a smokescreen. Regulations limiting midwifery were enacted more than 100 years ago, when birth outcomes were better for midwives than for physicians. Furthermore, competitors have a reason for banning lay midwives. Hospital births cost three times as much as home births assisted by a lay midwife (Anderson and Anderson 1999). As a result, lay midwives could claim a significant share of the market if allowed to practice without interference. This is about using the power of the state to eliminate a rival, not quality or safety."

"I think many licenses are scams designed to limit competition," said Kim, an advocate for lay midwives. "Licensure and similar rules keep incomes up, as Adam Smith pointed out in *The Wealth of Nations* in 1776. Whether it improves quality or protects consumers is debatable. We know that licensure boosts prices and practitioner incomes, but there's little evidence it does much else. Plus, state licensing boards usually get captured by the organizations they are supposed to be regulating. A better alternative would be certification. People who pass a state-run test could announce they are certified, and consumers could choose to patronize certified or uncertified providers."

Discussion questions:

- Would allowing lay midwives affect hospital prices or profits? Physician prices or profits?
- What is the argument for prohibiting practice without a license (as long as the absence of a license is disclosed)?
- Is there evidence that licensure improves quality?
- In medicine, licensure and certification coexist. Are there other fields in which certification and licensure coincide? Which seems to do a better job of protecting customers?
- How do licensure and certification differ in their protections for ill-informed consumers?
- Who controls the licensing boards for dentists, physicians, nurses, and other healthcare professions in your state? Is this jurisdiction consistent with Kim's claim that state licensing boards get captured?

on oneself) can be an effective competitive strategy. Most regulation of the health professions has been a result of this strategy because existing professionals have been grandfathered in and regulations apply only to newly licensed practitioners.

16.5 Regulatory Imperfections

When markets are not perfect, regulation can improve outcomes. For three reasons, however, regulation is likely to be equally imperfect: the need for decentralized decision making, conflicts between regulatory and financial incentives, and capture by regulated firms. Therefore, although new regulations can improve outcomes, there is no guarantee that they will.

Regulations work best when decision making is centralized and when "one size fits all." Healthcare does not fit these criteria. Patients' healthcare needs, preferences, and circumstances vary considerably, so decision making needs to be decentralized and individualized. In addition, regulatory and financial incentives need to be aligned to work well. When they are not, regulations are likely to be ignored or circumvented. For example, we know that healthcare organizations respond to financial incentives. If physicians find that treating patients in the hospital is more convenient than treating them in their offices, and there are no financial incentives to encourage outpatient care, utilization review (an analysis of patterns of care by an employer or insurer) is unlikely to reduce hospitalization rates.

Furthermore, the groups being regulated are likely to "capture" regulations based on even the most noble of intentions. *Capture* occurs when a group gains control of the administration of the regulations. Capture matters because the way the laws are implemented and enforced is as important as the laws themselves, and sooner or later the groups being regulated are likely to take control of the enforcement process. They will have better information than consumers, will pay more attention to the regulatory process than consumers, and will have a more intense interest in the regulatory process than consumers. Regulation does not eliminate consumers' rational ignorance (although regulations about disclosing information may reduce it). As a result, regulators are likely to be members of the regulated group or are likely to rely on members of the regulated group for advice. Compounding this dependence is the regulated group's ongoing interest in the regulations. Consumers and their advocates, in contrast, are likely to lose interest once the problems that led to the regulations have eased. Finally, the group being regulated typically has an intense interest in the outcome of the process, and most consumers do not. This disparity further increases the odds of capture because in the political arena, a small group

Case 16.2 **Self-Regulation**

"State pharmacy boards are too lax in their enforcement of the laws, too slow in innovating, and too prone to favor the interests of pharmacists. The public is often not represented on boards, and pharmacists are a majority of the board in every state," Angel said. "This is regulation for pharmacists, by pharmacists. If the safety of the public and the financial interests of the profession clash, the public will lose. Board members are almost always drawn from a list submitted by the state association of pharmacists. This is just another example of a profession using licensure to prevent competition, while talking about safety. For example, most pharmacists are opposed to periodic competency examinations. Concerns that some pharmacists might lose their licenses appear to outweigh concerns that there might be incompetent practitioners at work."

Discussion questions:
- Who sits on your state's board that regulates pharmacy, medicine, and dentistry? Are there any consumer representatives? Are members of the regulated profession a majority of the board?
- Could such boards function without representatives of the profession? Realistically, could a licensing board not be dominated by the profession in question?
- How would consumers be hurt if your state stopped licensing pharmacists and started certifying them instead? How would these two systems differ? Is this scenario an example of a result of regulatory capture? Can you suggest a strategy that would ensure that the licensing board would serve the public interest?
- Suppose your state stopped licensing pharmacists. Would hospitals replace high-paid pharmacists with untrained or minimally trained personnel? Would retail pharmacies replace high-paid pharmacists with untrained or minimally trained personnel? Explain your answers.

with an intense interest is likely to prevail over a larger group with more diffuse interests. As a result, regulation can best be described as "for the profession" rather than "of the profession."

16.6 Market Responses to Market Imperfections

Market responses to consumer ignorance can limit the need for regulation. Even imperfectly functioning markets incorporate incentives to serve consumers well. For most providers, repeat sales and customers are essential, so the incentives to meet customers' expectations are strong. Even when repeat customers are not major contributors to the business (as with a nursing home or plastic surgeon), the provider's reputation is one of its most important assets. Customers are not likely to detect profound agency problems. (See Chapter 12 for a fuller discussion of asymmetric information and agency.) Aware of their ineptitude for assessing poor performance, they often are willing to pay for information about quality and turn to consumer organizations (such as AARP) or information services (such as the National Committee for Quality Assurance) to aid them.

16.6.1 Tort and Contract Law

Tort law, which addresses compensation for a broad array of injuries, and *contract law*, which addresses breaches of agreement, can also remediate the shortcomings of healthcare markets. These legal remedies have powerful advantages. First, the threat of action is often enough to ensure compliance with explicit or implicit norms. If the probability of detecting noncompliance is high enough and the penalties are large enough, the threat of legal action will keep firms' behavior in check. Second, an agent's financial liability for nonperformance of a treatment usually exceeds the expected costs of the treatment, so tort and contract law create incentive for providers to perform. Aside from prompting legal costs, fines, and penalties, liability can damage the agent's reputation. Third, legal liability is outcome-oriented. Historically, regulation has focused on whether the structure of care and the processes of care comply with unverified norms, so its utility in matters of law is limited. Fourth, the legal system is more difficult to capture than most regulatory systems, especially when plaintiffs can take their cases to juries. Because consumers can initiate legal action themselves and because some lawyers are willing to accept the financial risks of failed suits by accepting contingency fees, access to legal remedies is more difficult to restrict than regulatory remedies.

Despite the power of tort and contract law, there also are disadvantages to their use. To begin, legal remedies are costly to apply. Because of the costs of bringing suit, consumers may face barriers when accessing the legal system. Second, consumer ignorance may compromise the effectiveness of legal remedies. If consumers do not realize that their bad outcome resulted from a breach of duty on the part of their provider, they will not bring suit. Alternatively, ignorant consumers may file suits when undesired outcomes resulted from bad luck, not negligence.

Absent a credible threat of being sued, incompetent or unscrupulous providers can continue unchecked. Even worse, the incentive for competent, scrupulous providers to invest resources in improving the quality of care may become diluted.

16.6.2 Information Dissemination

The legal system is both powerful and limited. First, it has limited physicians to areas in which they are competent, more effectively than state licensing boards. Medical licenses do not recognize differences in the skills of physicians. Were licenses the only guide, family practitioners would be able to perform neurosurgery. In fear of liability claims, hospitals also limit physicians to specific practices. Physicians, too, restrict their practices.

Second, studies of medical malpractice have shown that the majority of consumers who have suffered serious injuries as a result of negligence do not sue and receive no compensation. In addition, a high proportion of malpractice suits do not appear to involve provider negligence (Weiler et al. 1993). As a result, the malpractice system does not provide useful information on quality, and malpractice litigation's effect on the quality of care is not clear. In principle, publication of providers' malpractice histories should help consumers choose. Publication of risk-adjusted outcomes data would be better, as it would put pressure on organizations to improve quality and could reduce consumer ignorance.

16.6.3 Contracts

Contracts are a private regulatory system (albeit one that does not work when collective mechanisms for enforcing contracts do not function effectively). As with public regulations, contracts work best when financial and regulatory incentives are aligned. A contract that pays more for better performance will usually produce more satisfactory results than a contract that stipulates minimum performance requirements.

For example, modification of physicians' practice patterns is a challenge for physician organizations. Robinson (1999) notes that, under a pure capitation contract, physicians have financial incentives to avoid chronically ill patients, not to provide some types of care, and to refer large numbers of patients to other providers. Under a pure fee-for-service contract, in contrast, physicians have financial incentives to provide high volumes of billable services. Unfortunately, fee-for-service contracts also appear to result in fragmentation of care, upcoding, unbundling, and provision of services of questionable clinical value.

Many large practice organizations have responded by setting up contracts with physicians that blend capitation and fee-for-service payment. These contracts combine risk-adjusted capitation for basic primary care services, capitation stop-loss provisions that protect physicians from unexpectedly high costs, and fee-for-service payments for targeted services. These targeted services include vaccinations, visits to nursing facilities, and services that involve expensive supplies. The contracts also offer higher capitation rates for providers who provide a broader range of services. These contracts seek to change practice patterns by aligning the organization's and physicians' incentives.

Case 16.3   Changing Consumer Information

"Quality report cards are everywhere," said Kelly. "Some of the early efforts were real clunkers, but most look pretty sensible now. It makes sense to offer consumers information instead of protecting them from the consequences of their ignorance. A lot of the report cards emphasize clinical issues, but some look at courtesy and customer service. The advantages of report cards are immense. Physicians and patients get systematic information that helps them choose specialists and hospitals. Providers have an incentive to improve performance in areas they might have overlooked, and those who cannot compete are likely to drop out of the market. There is no downside. It may not even be necessary to set up elaborate pay-for-performance schemes. Fear of the fickle consumer may be incentive enough."

"While I like the idea of report cards," replied Lee, "there is little evidence that they have a significant impact. For example, an evaluation of the pay-for-performance pilot project that the Centers for Medicare & Medicaid Services launched in 2003 did not find that hospitals in the pilot improved more than other hospitals (Glickman et al. 2007). It's not that the hospitals in the pilot didn't improve. They did, but hospitals in the control group also got better. Study after study has found that report cards seem to have modest impacts on referrals and market share (Mukamel, Weimer, and Mushlin 2007). I like the idea of public reporting of price and quality data, but it's hard to make the case that report cards have had much of an effect."

"Whoa," replied Kelly, "I think you are getting confused. Most doctors and hospitals provide comparable levels of service. Only a few fall short of the mark. The goal is to improve population outcomes by steering patients away from those providers or getting the providers to improve. A few patient switches are enough to move market share, and I have a really hard time getting upset because we can't show clearly that report cards work because everyone is improving. Where we have report cards we see better performance. That's enough for me."

Discussion questions:

- What evidence can you find that report cards have improved quality?
- By what mechanisms could report cards improve reported market outcomes?
- Does the scarcity of scientific evidence on the effectiveness of report cards matter?
- Could publication of performance data be advantageous to hospitals or physicians?
- How do report cards address information asymmetries? Would reducing information asymmetries guarantee better markets?
- Does it matter whether report cards are produced by governments or private organizations?
- Why are a few patient switches enough to influence market outcomes?

16.7 Implications for Managers

Markets and regulations complement each other, as badly regulated markets will perform poorly. The usual reaction of managers is that less regulation is better than more, but this is not always true. For example, the regulations that govern the market for individual health insurance appear to drive up costs, make coverage difficult to buy, and decrease the value of policies for potential customers (Pollitz 2008). The primary value of insurance is that it reduces financial risks for its customers via pooling, but insurance regulations in most states make a variety of risk avoidance strategies very profitable for insurers. For example, insurers can limit their exposure to risk via rigorous underwriting, via exclusions, via post-claim underwriting, via restrictions on coverage, and via other mechanisms. Although these risk avoidance strategies may increase profits on existing customers, they reduce the value of individual plans for potential consumers. Not surprisingly, the market share of individual policies has steadily dropped in recent years (Buntin, Marquis, and Yegian 2004). With regulations better suited to the market, more individuals could buy coverage and insurers' profits could be higher.

Healthcare managers must understand the importance of regulations for their organizations and incorporate the effects of regulations in their decision making. Losses in the legislative or bureaucratic arenas may instigate regulations that put an organization at a significant disadvantage. Although it is tempting to see regulations as competitive tools, in practice their value is usually limited in competing with rivals in the same sector. Although zoning laws and certificate of need laws are notable exceptions, regulations usually apply the same rules for all the competitors in a sector.

Even when regulations could afford them a competitive advantage (perhaps by suppressing competition from rivals from other sectors), few organizations have the political strength and staying power to secure a long-lasting competitive advantage through political action. The exceptions tend to be large organizations that have a well-defined goal shared by all members, are well-funded, have a positive reputation, and advocate policies that benefit the public (although less influential interest groups often have the capacity to shape laws and subsequent regulations when the stakes are small for other groups). For most organizations the challenge will be to resist the creation of laws and administrative rulings that threaten to put them at a disadvantage. Fortunately, preventing change usually takes much less influence than does causing it.

The interests of healthcare providers appear to require more regulation than governments can be induced to develop. Nongovernmental regulation is widespread in healthcare. For example, certification of health plans and physicians grew out of the need to give customers more detailed information about quality than regulatory bodies could provide. This trend is likely to continue. Managers need to prepare their organizations to compete in environments in which competitive pressures force the release of detailed, audited information about costs and outcomes. Organizations that don't perform well, and are thus unable to attract well-informed customers, will fail.

16.8 Conclusion

Markets need a sound regulatory underpinning to secure property rights, define liability, create a mechanism for enforcing contracts, and constrain or sanction forms of competition. For example, Enthoven and Singer (1997) point out that for an insurance market to function effectively, it must have a mechanism for deciding when care is medically necessary. Such a mechanism benefits both insurers and patients. An insurer will lose sales if its contracts are too ambiguous because consumers will perceive the contracts' terms as meaningless. On the other hand, simple, rigid interpretations of medically necessary care would not take into account the diverse circumstances consumers face. Designing effective regulations is not easy. Even well-intentioned regulations can stifle innovation, and there is no guarantee that regulations will improve outcomes.

Homework

16.1   Why are many consumers apt to be rationally ignorant about their options?

16.2   Why would insurance coverage tend to increase rational ignorance?

16.3   A proposal has been advanced to limit advertising of pharmaceutical prices to prevent unfair pricing by national chains. You estimate that limits on price advertising will change the price elasticity of demand from –5.63 to –4.43. The marginal cost of a typical prescription is $40. A typical small pharmacy fills 25 prescriptions per day. A typical consumer fills 20 prescriptions per year. What will the economic effects of the limit be on consumers and pharmacists? Who is likely to be the more effective advocate for their position?

16.4   Prices for a medical procedure average $1,000 and range from $800 to $1,200. How much could a consumer paying full price save by getting the best price? Suppose that insurance is responsible for 75 percent of his spending and that his out-of-pocket spending is limited to $250. How much could he save by getting the best price?

16.5 Why are many economists opposed to licensure of medical facilities and personnel?

16.6 Identify circumstances in which there is both public and private regulation. Which serves consumers better? Why?

16.7 Find out who is on the board of the licensing agency for one of the health professions for your state. Are there more members of the profession being regulated or consumers on the board?

16.8 To reduce the costs of resolving insurance disputes, insurers have required that customers use arbitration. Arbitrators are required to be knowledgeable about medicine and insurance contracts. Why might you anticipate that the arbitration mechanism would wind up favoring the interests of the insurers?

16.9 How might the Food and Drug Administration be subject to capture? Who would be likely to capture the agency?

16.10 Hospital privileges usually restrict what physicians can do. Medical licenses do not. What drives this difference?

16.11 Consumers Union, the Leapfrog Group, and the Department of Health and Human Services have websites that provide consumer information about hospitals. Why are there multiple sources of information? Which of these sources did you find the most interesting?

16.12 Give an example of a healthcare product that is financed by the government but produced by private firms. Can you explain why this arrangement exists?

Chapter Glossary

Capture. Group takeover of regulations by which the group itself is regulated

Externality. A benefit or cost imposed on someone not a party to the transaction that caused it

Interest group model of regulation. Model that views regulations as attempts to further the interests of affected groups, usually producer groups

References

Anderson, R. E., and D. A. Anderson. 1999. "The Cost-Effectiveness of Home Birth." *Journal of Nurse Midwifery* 44 (1): 30–35.

Buntin, M., S. Marquis, and J. M. Yegian. 2004. "The Role of the Individual Health Insurance Market and Prospects for Change." *Health Affairs* 23 (6): 79–90.

Enthoven, A. C., and S. J. Singer. 1997. "Markets and Collective Action in Regulating Managed Care." *Health Affairs* 16 (6): 26–32.

Glickman, S. W., F. Ou, E. R. DeLong, M. T. Roe, B. L. Lytle, J. Mulgund, J. S. Rumsfeld, W. B. Gibler, E. M. Ohman, K. A. Schulman, and E. D. Peterson. 2007. "Pay for Performance, Quality of Care, and Outcomes in Acute Myocardial Infarction." *Journal of the American Medical Association* 297 (21): 2373–80.

Johnson, K. C., and B. A. Daviss. 2005. "Outcomes of Planned Home Births with Certified Professional Midwives: A Large Prospective Study in North America." *British Medical Journal* 330 (7505): 1416–23.

Mukamel, D. B., D. L. Weimer, and A. I. Mushlin. 2007. "Interpreting Market Share Changes as Evidence for Effectiveness of Quality Report Cards." *Medical Care* 45 (12): 1227–32.

Pollitz, K. 2008. "Private Health Insurance Market Regulation." [Online information; retrieved 2/2/09.] http://finance.senate.gov/healthsummit2008/Statements/Karen%20Pollitz%20Testimony.pdf.

Robinson, J. C. 1999. "Blended Payment Methods in Physician Organizations Under Managed Care." *Journal of the American Medical Association* 282 (13): 1258–63.

U.S. Department of Justice. 2000. "Brief for the United States and the Federal Trade Commission as Amici Curiae." [Online information; retrieved 2/3/09.] www.usdoj.gov/atr/cases/f230700/230741.htm.

Weiler, P. C., H. H. Hiatt, J. P. Newhouse, W. G. Johnson, T. A. Brennan, and L. L. Leape. 1993. *A Measure of Malpractice: Medical Injury, Malpractice Litigation, and Patient Compensation.* Cambridge, MA: Harvard University Press.

STRATEGIC BEHAVIOR

After reading this chapter, students will be able to:

- **define** Nash equilibrium,
- **apply** game theory concepts to simple strategic situations,
- **explain** why it is important to understand your rivals' options, and
- **discuss** the application of game theory to healthcare management.

- Strategic thinking is vital for most healthcare managers.
- Strategic thinking is essential in negotiating contracts.
- A clear understanding of your best option without a deal is key to successful negotiation.
- Strategic thinking is essential in responding to initiatives by large rivals.
- Knowing your options and your rivals' options is fundamental to strategic thinking.
- A dominant strategy is one a firm should pursue no matter what its rival does.
- In a Nash equilibrium, none of the players want to change their strategy because the strategy of the other players keeps a change from being advantageous.
- Players can alter the outcomes of games by making credible threats or commitments.

17.1 Introduction

Strategic thinking is vital for most healthcare managers. In any market, managers routinely negotiate contracts with other companies. In some markets, skillful responses to the strategies of rivals are part of successful leadership. In healthcare markets, the quest for market power and economies of scale limits the number of competitors. In such an oligopolistic market, managers must ask, "If my rivals act effectively to realize their goals, how should I incorporate their expected behavior into my decision making?"

Managers may use game theory to answer this question. To understand a game, consider each option open to a player and then identify the rival's best response to each option. Then identify the player's best response for each of the rival's options. Game theory shows that even simple strategy problems can have complex solutions. Sometimes formal analysis will not help. But in other cases, it will make clear your best response to your rivals' strategies and even how to influence what your rivals do.

Competing against a well-organized, aggressive rival is difficult. But this challenge confronts many healthcare managers. In any market with only a few players, each competitor must track what the others are doing. For instance, an insurance company's sales will be affected by a competitor's introduction of a new product. Especially in markets where growth is slow, failure to respond to the initiatives of rivals can be damaging.

Game theory recognizes two types of games. In *cooperative games*, the players can negotiate binding contracts. Managers need to understand the bargaining process that leads to efficient contracts and when a contract can be binding. Players in *noncooperative games* cannot negotiate binding contracts, but must "play" against one another. Noncooperative games resemble recreational games like checkers, poker, and backgammon. Each player acts to further his or her own interests, and the more skillful player wins. Market competition differs from checkers, poker, and backgammon in that the resources available to each player can vary. "Winning" against a rival with more resources and lower costs may involve identifying a market niche where your rival's strengths are negated.

17.2 Cooperative Games

Bargaining is the hallmark of cooperative games. Perhaps the most valuable asset in bargaining is an understanding of the worst deal you will accept and the worst deal the other side will accept. Failure to agree is always a possibility, and both sides need to gain from the bargain. Parties seldom agree to terms that are worse than their "no deal" option. Research confirms that playing fair is also important. Negotiators may not agree to deals they regard as unfair, even a deal that is better than their "no deal" option. Most negotiators will interact over and over, and even when this is not true, a bargainer's reputation becomes known. Unless it is advantageous to develop a reputation for being difficult to do business with, being known for reliability and honesty will make bargaining easier and more rewarding. Taking advantage of a partner's inexperience or lack of information is a bad idea. Good managers treasure their reputations, realizing opponents' belief in their good faith is a valuable asset (Shister 1997).

The gains from bargaining need not be distributed equally. One party may have better options or less to lose if negotiations break down. The art of negotiation is to press this advantage just far enough and no further. If the stronger party presses its advantage, it risks creating an enemy. On the other hand, a party in a weak negotiating position should not expect to share equally in the rewards of an agreement.

Negotiation is involved in contracts with suppliers, sales to customers, agreements with partners, deals with peers, and arrangements with subordinates. Yet many managers do not think systematically about these negotiations (Ertel 1999). They assume negotiation is always a *zero-sum game*, in which one party's gains equal another party's losses. This is not always true. Some negotiations can result in gains for all parties.

Most business relationships are long term, so a natural consideration is whether a negotiation strengthened or weakened the relationship between the parties. From there three questions arise about how the bargaining process affected the relationship: Did the negotiation allow the parties to converse about problem solving? Did the negotiation explore innovations that might let all parties win? Did the negotiation advance the interests of all parties? Of course, if these criteria are to matter, they must be the criteria that drive the incentives—bonuses, commissions, promotions, or nonfinancial rewards—negotiators face. Otherwise, the criteria will be just rhetoric.

Negotiators may seek to change the game by proposing alternatives. For example, a supply firm that allows just-in-time ordering reduces inventory and acquisition costs for its customer. At the same time, just-in-time ordering makes other vendors less competitive, so the bargaining process puts less pressure on margins.

If bargaining does not result in a contract that benefits both parties, it makes no sense to sign. By the same token, unless it is in your partner's interest to carry out the agreement you have crafted, it is a bad agreement. Contracts need to be enforceable, and at low cost. An agreement that forces your partner to do something against his will is likely to fail. Taking legal action to enforce a contract or keeping the bond your partner has posted generally means you have not gotten what you wanted. An enforceable contract is one both partners want to live up to. An important negotiation skill is the ability to write a contract neither party wants to breach.

Case 17.1   **Negotiating with Athena**

"Okay, we are getting 105 percent of Medicare fees from Athena," said Jordan Crosby. "That's not so hot, but I have other concerns about this contract. Emerson has done some analysis that suggests Athena is a minor player for us and that we've had difficulty getting paid in a timely fashion. Only about 4 percent of our patients are covered by Athena, and over 20 percent of our claims with them are not getting paid within 30 days."

"I've worked with a consultant for the last three months," said Emerson Robertson, executive director. "She says the Athena rates are a little below the prevailing rates in the market. Most of the smaller PPOs are paying about 110 percent of Medicare, and most are paying virtually all their clean claims within 30 days. Now Blue Cross is paying about 104 percent of Medicare rates, but it has a 53 percent market share. I think we can do better than this with Athena. Its proposal is for 'fees equal to 100 percent of the Athena fee schedule' and a '0.5 percent interest payment per month for all clean claims more than 30 days old.' The law here is that 'there shall be added to any undisputed service claim form which is not paid within 25 working days an amount equal to 10 percent of the unpaid balance,' so Athena is asking us to waive rights we have under state law."

Discussion questions:
- What is the worst deal this practice will accept?
- Is the practice in a weak or strong position in its negotiations with Athena?
- Is this a zero-sum game?
- Does a win for the practice rule out a win for Athena?
- How can the concerns of the practice be presented as solving problems for Athena?
- The practice is clearly in a better negotiating posture as a result of analyzing data on its relationship with Athena and on the market as a whole. What additional information should Emerson review before starting negotiations?

17.3 Noncooperative Games

Cooperative games are complex, but noncooperative games are far more complex, because neither the rules nor the agreements are written down. When competing in oligopoly markets, managers need to focus on five key issues:

1. knowing your options,
2. knowing your rival's options,
3. understanding your rival's point of view,

4. forecasting your rival's responses to your initiatives or changes in the market, and
5. influencing your rival's responses.

All of these are important, but understanding your options is by far the most important. If you have not thought of a strategy, you will not pursue it. If you have not seen that a strategy is impractical, you may waste time trying to implement it.

17.4 Dominant Strategies

Is there a dominant strategy? That is, will my best strategy be the same no matter what my rival does? Will my rival's best strategy be the same no matter what I do? In Figure 17.1, Bethany has a dominant strategy. No matter what Avalon does, Bethany should accept the PPO contract. (Avalon's choices are listed along the left side of the table, and Bethany's choices are listed along the top of the table.) If Avalon joins the PPO, Bethany will earn $200 if it joins and $100 if it does not. If Avalon does not join the PPO, Bethany will earn $450 if it joins and only $400 if it does not. This makes planning much simpler for the managers of Avalon. They need only choose the best strategy given the fact that Bethany will join no matter what. In this instance, Avalon should also join the PPO. Note, though, that Avalon does not have a dominant strategy. Its best strategy depends on Bethany's strategy.

Figure 17.1 is a payoff matrix. A *payoff matrix* is an attempt to list each player's possible strategies and forecast the gain (or payoff) each will realize. For example, Figure 17.1 predicts Avalon will get a payoff of $400 and Bethany will get a payoff of $200 if both accept the PPO contract. Obviously the payoff forecasts are conjectures, but they need not be precise to be helpful. For example, Figure 17.1 reflects three simple rules. First, joining the PPO reduces prices and profits, with two significant exceptions. Second, a firm whose rival has joined the PPO can increase market share and profits by also joining. Third, Bethany has enough excess capacity that its

FIGURE 17.1

Accepting a PPO Contract as a Dominant Strategy

	Bethany	
	Accept PPO Contract	*Refuse PPO Contract*
Avalon **Accept PPO Contract**	$Y_A = 400, Y_B = 200$	$Y_A = 600, Y_B = 100$
Avalon **Refuse PPO Contract**	$Y_A = 100, Y_B = 450$	$Y_A = 700, Y_B = 400$

Sidebar 17.1 Playing Games in Memphis

In 1988, Baptist Memorial Hospital and Methodist Hospitals of Memphis submitted certificate of need applications to the Tennessee Health Facilities Commission to authorize the purchase of positron emission tomography (PET) equipment. The Commission approved both applications, but neither hospital actually purchased the equipment. Three years later, the two hospitals signed a joint venture agreement to provide PET, but the joint venture did not purchase the PET equipment. The explanation for this odd sequence of events lies in strategic considerations (Weingarten 1999).

Interviews with senior managers confirmed that Baptist and Methodist proceeded with PET certificate of need applications mainly to preempt each other. Neither had much confidence that PET would be very profitable. Many insurers did not cover it, and demand forecasts were nebulous. Even more important, neither manager was responding to concerted advocacy by physicians. Given PET's high cost, delay seemed the logical decision, yet neither wanted the other hospital to be the recipient of the sole certificate of need.

When the Commission unexpectedly granted both certificates of need, a new preemption strategy was needed. The joint venture was a creative way to ensure that neither would be left without PET, if it should become standard in tertiary radiology. It prevented either partner from proceeding independently. Neither was concerned about other hospitals, since there were no plausible alternative PET providers in Memphis. The joint venture also represented an option on the technology. As equipment prices fell and PET became more widely accepted, the hospitals were positioned to proceed. They had converted the noncooperative preemption game in which both were likely to suffer losses into a cooperative game in which neither stood to lose.

It is interesting to note that there were no PET scanners in Memphis until 2000. By 2002 there were six. By then the annual cost of a PET scanner had fallen by a third, and it was covered for a variety of uses by Medicare and many commercial insurers (Berger, Gould, and Barnett 2003).

profits will rise if it joins the PPO and Avalon does not. Any set of payoffs that follows the same rules would force the same conclusions. The fact that your forecasts are guesstimates does not reduce the value of a payoff matrix. Simply writing down your options and your rival's options can clarify the situation quite a bit. It also allows others to add options you haven't considered or to critique your assumptions about payoffs. It may then become obvious what your rival is going to do or what you should do.

The game in Figure 17.1 has an *equilibrium* outcome. Once both have accepted the PPO contract, neither will want to defect. If either player dropped out of the PPO (and the other player did not), the income of the player who dropped out would fall. This type of strategic equilibrium is called a *Nash equilibrium*. This equilibrium will persist even though both firms would prefer an environment in which neither of them accepted the PPO contract. Both of them refusing to sign is not an equilibrium, however, because Bethany has an incentive to defect from that situation: Its income is highest when it accepts the PPO contract and Avalon does not.

Games in which the outcome that both parties prefer is not an equilibrium are called *prisoner's dilemmas*. The name comes from a game in which two prisoners are questioned separately. Each is promised a reduced sentence for testifying against the other. If one testifies, the other receives a long sentence. If neither testifies, neither is convicted and both go free. The promise of a reduced sentence induces both to confess, so both draw long sentences. Managers do not want to play a prisoner's dilemma game, but there are ways to avoid them.

17.5 Games Without Dominant Strategies

Small changes in market conditions can lead to very different outcomes. Only one number has changed between Figures 17.1 and 17.2. Bethany's income is forecast to be only $350 when it accepts the PPO contract and Avalon does not. Refusing the contract gives Bethany a forecast income of $400, which means accepting the PPO contract is no longer a dominant strategy for Bethany. It also means this game has two possible Nash equilibria: both accepting or both refusing.

This example illustrates two important features of strategic behavior. First, contests can have many different outcomes, and managers may prefer some of them to others. Second, by changing payoffs managers can change the outcomes of games.

A classic type of game with multiple equilibria is a *coordination game*. In a coordination game, everyone wins if all of the parties agree to certain norms or standards. Since Avalon and Bethany are in the same town and often serve the same customers, there are significant advantages to using the same electronic health record (EHR). Both will be able to reduce costs and improve care. Furthermore, each electronic health record will become more

FIGURE 17.2

A Game with No Dominant Strategy

	Bethany	
	Accept PPO Contract	*Refuse PPO Contract*
Avalon *Accept PPO Contract*	$Y_A = 400, Y_B = 200$	$Y_A = 600, Y_B = 100$
Refuse PPO Contract	$Y_A = 100, Y_B = 350$	$Y_A = 700, Y_B = 400$

FIGURE 17.3
A Coordination
Game

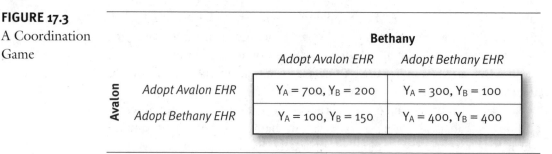

		Bethany	
		Adopt Avalon EHR	Adopt Bethany EHR
Avalon	Adopt Avalon EHR	$Y_A = 700, Y_B = 200$	$Y_A = 300, Y_B = 100$
	Adopt Bethany EHR	$Y_A = 100, Y_B = 150$	$Y_A = 400, Y_B = 400$

valuable if the other hospital also uses it. Figure 17.3 depicts a situation in which both parties using the same electronic health record (either Avalon's or Bethany's) is an equilibrium. The problem is that each strongly prefers its own electronic health record be the standard. Coordination games help us understand why standard setting is so common and so contentious. For example, Health Level Seven is a voluntary, not-for-profit organization that helps develop international healthcare standards. The organization and its members set standards for exchanging, integrating, sharing, and retrieving electronic health information. The difficulty is that some vendors of electronic health records adhere to other standards. While all agree on the need for common standards, there is controversy about what the standards should be.

17.6 Repeated Games

Most business relationships are long term. This can fundamentally change the winning strategy. As the old saying goes, "Fool me once, shame on you. Fool me twice, shame on me." When players (organizations or individuals) interact repeatedly, the range of sensible strategies expands. Threats of future retribution may circumvent aggressive price competition, or a player's reputation may costlessly deter entry by rivals.

Figure 17.4 describes the payoffs for a game involving entry. Universal already provides managed behavioral health services in a local market. It is the only significant player and realizes handsome profits. The managers of Global must assess whether they should enter this market. If they predict, based on its behavior in other markets, that Universal will not start a price war, Global will enter the market. Its profits will be 200, because Universal will share the market. Universal may threaten a price war, but that is not a credible threat, as the best thing for Universal to do if Global enters is to avoid a price war. After all, Universal will lose $5 if it starts a price war and earn $200 if it does not. The managers of Global assume that there will be downward pressure on prices, even if Universal does not start a price war.

Suppose, on the other hand, Universal recognizes that the only way for its high profits to continue is to develop a reputation as an irrational com-

FIGURE 17.4
Universal Is a
Rational
Incumbent

	Global	
	Enter Market	*Do Not Enter Market*
Universal — *Share the Market*	$Y_U = 200, Y_G = 200$	$Y_U = 600, Y_G = 0$
Universal — *Start a Price War*	$Y_U = -5, Y_G = -5$	$Y_U = 400, Y_G = 0$

petitor. It makes it known that it evaluates its regional managers primarily in terms of market share and only secondarily in terms of profits. A manager who delivers high profits gets bonuses, but a manager who loses market share gets fired. So Global or any other competitor must recognize that Universal's regional managers will defend market share with a passion. Indeed, Figure 17.5 illustrates a situation in which one of Universal's regional managers has expanded capacity and cut prices preemptively. This reduces profits whether Global enters the market or not, but it makes it sensible for this manager to start a price war if Global enters. Universal need not do this in every market. Its real goal is to broadcast a credible message that it will take unreasonable steps to protect market share. Knowing that Universal is an irrational competitor, Global will not want to enter markets in which Universal is a player. Of course, Universal may have to launch a vigorous price war when a rival does enter, just to reiterate that it means business.

Both Universal and its rivals understand that the most profitable outcome will result from Universal merely appearing irrational. This will deter most prospective rivals, although the price war that follows entry is quite costly.

17.7 Credible Threats and Commitments

A *credible threat* is a strategy that punishes your opponent while being your best response to your rival's action. In Figure 17.6, Avalon makes an incredible threat to join an HMO if Bethany enters the market. The threat is not

FIGURE 17.5
Universal Is an
Irrational
Incumbent

	Global	
	Enter Market	*Do Not Enter Market*
Universal — *Share the Market*	$Y_U = -20, Y_G = 200$	$Y_U = 600, Y_G = 0$
Universal — *Start a Price War*	$Y_U = -5, Y_G = -5$	$Y_U = 400, Y_G = 0$

Case 17.2   **Bidding for North Shore Clinics**

"North Shore has just announced its intention to close. It plans to end patient care operations at the hospital and sell its clinics in Beech Wood, Forest Hills, and Knoxville. The hospital is a 212-bed facility that was built in 1974. Its physical plant is badly dated and had only 52 percent occupancy. It was steadily losing money and had no realistic prospect of turning itself around. The clinics, while not profitable and not operating at full capacity, still generated 203,000 visits per year, many from established, insured patients. So," said Parker Quinn, "I assume we are interested. This could be a chance for Smith Memorial to capture significant market share."

"Do we bid? If so, how much do we bid?" asked Alexis Rogers. "The hospital is not really worth anything as a going concern, but the land has value. The site is probably worth $12 million to $25 million. We should be able to resell it within a year. The Beech Wood Clinic is probably worth $6 million to $12 million; the Forest Hills Clinic is probably worth $8 million to $15 million; and the Knoxville Clinic is probably worth $4 million to $10 million."

"So, somewhere between $30 million and $62 million is the answer? I love how you finance people can be so precise," said Elliot Jefferson, CEO of Smith Memorial. "But actually, we only need to offer $1 more than Central Health. Are they bidding? What will they offer? Will anyone else be bidding? Will North Shore accept bids for parts of the property? We only want the Forest Hills Clinic and Knoxville Clinic. The Beech Wood Clinic is too close to our East Side Clinic to be of much use to us."

credible because if Bethany enters the market, Avalon's best response will be to refuse to join the HMO. So, even though Avalon can punish Bethany for entering the market, Bethany will ignore the threat.

Avalon can force Bethany to respect its threat by changing its circumstances. For example, Avalon can build enough capacity to make joining the HMO its best strategy if Bethany enters the market. Given the situation in Figure 17.7, Bethany would be wise to respect Avalon's threat, because if

FIGURE 17.6

Avalon's Threat to Join the HMO if Bethany Enters the Market Is Not Credible

		Bethany	
		Enter Market	*Do Not Enter Market*
Avalon	*Join HMO*	$Y_A = 300, Y_B = -10$	$Y_A = 600, Y_B = 0$
	Do Not Join HMO	$Y_A = 400, Y_B = 300$	$Y_A = 700, Y_B = 0$

"Well," replied Alexis, "North Shore has made it clear that it will demand bids for all of the properties in the first round. If none of the bids exceeds its undisclosed reservation price, it will look for bids for individual properties. I am positive Central Health will bid, if only because it knows we want Forest Hills and Knoxville. It really wants Beech Wood and would like to have Forest Hills. You know, we have already developed plans to build clinics that fit our specifications on bus lines with parking in Forest Hills and Knoxville. Our estimates are that we will be able to take occupancy in 14 months at a total cost of $18 million. Plus, I have heard that North West Properties really wants the hospital site. It plans to turn it into retail and apartments. It thinks $20 million will buy the property."

Discussion questions:
- Should Smith Memorial bid for the North Shore assets? What is the most it will bid? How did you calculate this?
- Will Central Health bid? What is the most it will bid? How did you calculate this?
- Elliott Jefferson seems to believe no one else will be bidding for the North Shore assets. How would your answers be different if there were a bidder that planned to reopen the hospital and keep all the clinics?
- How would your answers be different if Central Health could not bid?
- Suppose that Smith Memorial, Central Health, and North West Properties formed a partnership to bid on the North Shore assets. How much would the partnership bid?

Bethany enters the market, Avalon has no choice but to join the HMO. That being the case, Bethany will not want to enter.

Recall that in our initial example of a noncooperative game, accepting a PPO contract was a dominant strategy for Bethany. (Figure 17.8 reproduces that example.) Bethany has an incentive to defect from the refuse/refuse outcome, and neither player has an incentive to defect from the accept/accept outcome.

		Bethany	
		Enter Market	*Do Not Enter Market*
Avalon	*Join HMO*	$Y_A = 200, Y_B = -10$	$Y_A = 600, Y_B = 0$
	Do Not Join HMO	$Y_A = 100, Y_B = 300$	$Y_A = 600, Y_B = 0$

FIGURE 17.7

Avalon's Threat to Join the HMO if Bethany Enters the Market Is Credible

FIGURE 17.8
Accepting a
PPO Contract
as a Dominant
Strategy

		Bethany	
		Accept PPO Contract	*Refuse PPO Contract*
Avalon *Accept PPO Contract*		$Y_A = 400, Y_B = 200$	$Y_A = 600, Y_B = 100$
Refuse PPO Contract		$Y_A = 100, Y_B = 450$	$Y_A = 700, Y_B = 400$

As the only two players in a continuously repeating game, Avalon and Bethany might be able to monitor cheating and successfully avoid accepting the PPO contract (or sign, but offer little or no discount). A simple tit-for-tat strategy might work. In such a strategy, Bethany would make clear its plan to refuse the PPO contract unless Avalon accepted, in which case it would join as well and profits would fall for both. As long as both parties expect to play indefinitely and do not expect entry by other organizations, this simple strategy might well support a refuse/refuse equilibrium. Neither would want to defect because of the long-term consequences.

If there were more players, however, one player would eventually offer discounts to gain market share. Or, if entry were possible, at some point someone would conclude that the system of tacit cooperation was about to break down and would defect. With many rivals or with easy entry, tacit cooperation is almost sure to break down. When it does, price competition becomes the norm and margins get squeezed. Of course, individual organizations can still try to gain higher markups by differentiating their products.

17.8 Conclusions

In a market with only a few participants, firms recognize their mutual interdependence. The best strategy for one player depends on the strategies the others choose. Each needs to be concerned with what its rivals are doing, hence each must watch its rivals carefully and predict their next moves. Because of this interdependence, oligopolists face a complex decision-making process. Each must determine its best response to its opponents' possible strategies and deduce what it should do in reaction.

Equilibrium in an oligopoly market occurs when each participant chooses to maintain its current strategy, given what the other participants are doing. In other words, it is in each firm's self-interest to keep production quantities or prices at the equilibrium level.

The game of business competition can be quite complex. Nonetheless, five keys stand out: Know your options. Know your rival's options. Understand your rival's point of view. Forecast your rival's responses to changed circumstances. Influence your rival's responses via credible threats.

Homework

17.1 Two pediatric groups must choose either a low-cost, low-amenity strategy, L, or a high-cost, high-amenity strategy, H. In the table below, identify any Nash equilibria and the cooperative outcome. Which group would benefit most from cooperation? (The first number in each cell is the per-MD income in group 1.)

		Group 2	
		H	*L*
Group 1	*H*	58, 57	150, 130
	L	70, 140	65, 65

17.2 Two makers of allergy drugs, firms A and B, expect to compete for a number of years. At present, both firms have small marketing budgets and high profits. What marketing expenditures might the companies be considering? What are the possible equilibrium strategies? How could the game be changed legally to the advantage of the firms? Set the payoff matrix up with A's actions defining the rows and B's actions defining the columns. In each cell, A's payoff should be listed first. If firm A increases its marketing budget and B does too, A will earn \$30 and B will earn \$25. If firm A increases its marketing budget and B does not, A will earn \$70 and B will earn \$35. If firm A keeps its marketing budget small and B does too, A and B will each earn \$65. If firm A keeps its marketing budget small and B increases its marketing, A will earn \$40 and B will earn \$70.

17.3 How do cooperative and noncooperative games differ? Give a healthcare example of each.

17.4 Why is it important to reach mutually advantageous agreements? Can you think of an example in which bargaining was not a zero-sum game?

17.5 What's a dominant strategy? Can you think of a dominant strategy for healthcare firms?

17.6 Scythian and Galacian must make sealed bids to a PPO. Explain why Scythian and Galacian will wind up in the low price/low price equilibrium, even though both would be better off in the high price/high price equilibrium. The table below reports the profits for the two firms for each cell of the strategy matrix.

		Scythian	
		Low Price	*High Price*
Galacian	*Low Price*	G = 25, S = 25	G = 250, S = −125
	High Price	G = −125, S = 250	G = 125, S = 125

17.7 Suppose Galacian announced it would submit a high price bid before the bidding closed. Would that change the outcome?

17.8 Suppliers routinely provide materials on credit to buyers. The materials are perishable and can be resold, yet suppliers often have little protection against a dishonest buyer. Explain why buyers do not often take advantage of suppliers.

17.9 The average salary for pediatricians who have just finished residency is $150,000. One of the residents at a nearby hospital has a sick child and will have to stay in town for at least a year. The resident was forced to turn down several out-of-town offers. The resident's best current offer is a $40,000 part-time job in a free clinic. The resident is your top candidate, and no other local openings seem likely. What salary should you offer? Why?

17.10 You own a pharmacy. A competitor launches a "We Will Not Be Undersold" campaign, promising to give customers 150 percent of any difference between its prices and the advertised prices of other pharmacies. How should you react?

17.11 Akron and Bethesda medical centers compete with each other. Bethesda has a larger network but is relatively inefficient. Akron has a small network of clinics but is contemplating either fast or slow expansion. Bethesda is contemplating a major investment in continuous quality improvement (CQI) to improve its quality of care and lower its costs. Does either have a dominant strategy? What implications does that have for the other? Akron's profits are the first entry in each cell; Bethesda's are the second.

		Bethesda	
		CQI	*No CQI*
Akron	*Fast*	A = 58, B = 157	A = 150, B = 130
	Slow	A = 70, B = 140	A = 65, B = 65

Chapter Glossary

Cooperative game. A game in which the players can negotiate binding contracts

Dominant strategy. A strategy that is advantageous to pursue no matter what rivals do

Game theory. The analysis of strategies when rivals may anticipate one another's actions

Nash equilibrium. A situation in which none of the participants want to change strategies, given what the others are doing

Noncooperative game. A game in which the players cannot negotiate binding contracts

Prisoner's dilemma. A game in which the outcome both parties prefer is not an equilibrium

Zero-sum game. A game in which any gains by one player must be matched by losses by another player

References

Berger, M., M. K. Gould, and P. G. Barnett. 2003. "The Cost of Positron Emission Tomography in Six United States Veterans Affairs Hospitals and Two Academic Medical Centers." *American Journal of Roentgenology* 181 (2): 359–65.

Ertel, D. 1999. "Turning Negotiation into a Corporate Capability." *Harvard Business Review* 77 (3): 55–70.

Shister, N. 1997. *10-Minute Guide to Negotiating*. New York: Macmillan Spectrum.

Weingarten, J. P. 1999. "Cooperative Ventures in a Competitive Environment: The Influence of Regulation on Management Decisions." *Journal of Healthcare Management* 44 (4): 282–300.

GLOSSARY

Adverse selection. The willingness of high-risk consumers to pay more for insurance than low-risk consumers (Organizations that have difficulty distinguishing high-risk from low-risk consumers are unlikely to be profitable.)

Agency. An arrangement in which one person (the agent) takes actions on behalf of another (the principal).

Arc elasticity. An elasticity calculation that uses the average of the data to calculate percentage changes.

Asymmetric information. Information known to one party in a transaction but not another.

Attribute-based product differentiation. Making customers aware of differences among products.

Average cost. Total cost divided by total output.

Capitation. Payment per person. (The payment does not depend on the services provided.)

Capture. Group takeover of regulations by which the group itself is regulated.

Case-based payment. A single payment for an episode of care. (The payment does not change if fewer services or more services are provided.)

Coinsurance. A form of cost sharing in which a patient pays a share of the bill rather than a set fee.

Complement. A product used in conjunction with another product.

Cooperative game. A game in which the players can negotiate binding contracts.

Copayment. A fee the patient must pay in addition to the amount paid by insurance.

Cost. The value of a resource in its next best use.

Cost-benefit analysis. An analysis that compares the value of an innovation with its costs. Value is measured as willingness to pay for the innovation or willingness to accept compensation to allow it to be implemented.

Cost-effectiveness analysis. An analysis that measures the cost of an innovation per unit of change in a single outcome.

Cost-minimization analysis. An analysis that measures the cost of two or more innovations with the same patient outcomes.

Cost sharing. The general term for direct payments to providers by insurance beneficiaries. (Deductibles, copayments, and coinsurance are forms of cost sharing.)

Cost shifting. The hypothesis that price differences are due to efforts by providers to make up for losses in some lines of business by charging higher prices in other lines of business.

Cost-utility analysis. An analysis that measures the cost of an innovation per quality-adjusted life year.

Cross-price elasticity. The percentage change in the quantity demanded associated with a 1 percent change in the price of a related product.

Decision tree. A visual decision support tool that depicts the values and probabilities of the outcomes of a choice.

Demand. The amounts of a good or service that will be purchased at different prices when all other factors are held constant.

Demand curve. A tool for describing how much consumers are willing to buy at different prices.

Demand shift. A shift that occurs when a factor other than price (e.g., consumer incomes) changes.

Diagnosis-related groups (DRGs). Case groups that underlie Medicare's case-based payment system for hospitals.

Discounting. Adjusting the value of future costs and benefits to reflect the willingness of consumers to trade current consumption for future consumption. Usually future values are discounted by $1/(1 + r)^n$, with r the discount rate and n the number of periods in the future the cost or benefit will be realized.

Dominant strategy. A strategy that is advantageous to pursue no matter what rivals do.

Economies of scale. When larger organizations have lower average costs.

Economies of scope. When multiproduct organizations have lower average costs.

Efficient. Productive of the most valuable output possible, given its inputs. (Viewed differently, an efficient organization uses the least expensive inputs possible, given the quality and quantity of output it produces.)

Elastic. A term used to describe demand when the quantity demanded falls by more than 1 percent when the price rises by 1 percent. This term is usually applied only to price elasticities of demand.

Elasticity. The percent change in a dependent variable associated with a 1 percent change in an independent variable.

Equilibrium price. Price at which the quantity demanded equals the quantity supplied. (There is no shortage or surplus.)

Expected value. The sum of the probability of each possible outcome multiplied by the value of the outcome.

Exponential moving average. An average that gives decreasing weight to older data. For example, a common formula is $\hat{x}_t = \alpha \hat{x}_{t-1} + (1 - \alpha) x_{t-1}$, which gives less and less weight over time to the observations that produced $\hat{x}_{t-1}$.

External benefit. A positive impact of a transaction for a consumer or producer not involved in the transaction.

External cost. A negative impact of a transaction for a consumer or producer not involved in the transaction.

Externality. A benefit or cost imposed on someone who is not a party to the transaction that causes it.

Factor of production. Another name for an input.

Fee-for-service. An insurance plan that pays providers on the basis of their charges for services.

Fixed costs. Costs that do not vary according to output.

Formulary. A formulary can be a list of drugs routinely used by a healthcare provider or it can be a list of prescription drugs covered by insurance.

Free rider. Someone who benefits from a public good without bearing its cost.

Gain sharing. A general strategy for rewarding those who contribute to an organization's success. (Profit sharing is one form of gain sharing. Rewards can be based on other criteria as well.)

Game theory. The analysis of strategies when rivals may anticipate one another's actions.

Group model HMO. HMO that contracts with a physician group to provide services.

Health maintenance organization (HMO). A firm that provides comprehensive healthcare benefits to enrollees in exchange for a premium. (Originally, HMOs were distinct from other insurance firms because providers were not paid on a fee-for-service basis and because enrollees faced no cost-sharing requirements.)

Income elasticity of demand. The percent change in the quantity demanded associated with a 1 percent increase in income.

Increase or decrease in demand. A shift in the entire list of amounts that will be purchased at different prices.

Incremental. A small change from the current situation.

Inelastic. A term used to describe demand when the quantity demanded falls by less than 1 percent when the price rises by 1 percent. This term is usually applied only to price elasticities of demand.

Input. A good or service used in the production of another good or service.

Interest group model of regulation. Model that views regulations as attempts to further the interests of affected groups, usually producer groups.

Life year. One additional year of life. (A life year can also represent 1/nth of a year of life for n people.)

Limit pricing. Setting prices low enough to discourage entry into a market.

Managed care. A loosely defined term that includes PPO and HMO plans, sometimes used to describe the techniques insurance companies use.

Marginal. A small change from the current situation.

Marginal analysis. Assessment of the effects of small changes in a decision variable (such as price or the volume of output) on outcomes (such as costs, profits, or the probability of recovery).

Marginal cost pricing. The use of information about marginal costs and the price elasticity of demand to set profit-maximizing prices.

Marginal or incremental cost. The cost of producing an additional unit of output.

Marginal revenue. The revenue from selling an additional unit of output.

Market demand. The sum of the demands of all consumers in a market.

Market system. A system that uses prices to ration goods and services.

Mean absolute deviation. The average absolute difference between a forecast and the actual value. It is absolute because it converts both 9 and –9 to 9. The Excel function = abs() performs this conversion.

Medicaid. The name given to a collection of state programs that meet standards set by the Centers for Medicare & Medicaid Services but are run by state agencies. (Medicaid serves those with incomes low enough to qualify for their state's program.)

Medicare. An insurance program for the elderly and disabled that is run by the Centers for Medicare & Medicaid Services.

Medicare Part A. Coverage for inpatient hospital, skilled nursing, hospice, and home health care services.

Medicare Part B. Coverage for outpatient services and medical equipment.

Monopolist. A firm with no rivals.

Monopolistic competitor. A competitor with multiple rivals whose products are imperfect substitutes.

Moral hazard. The incentive to use additional care that having insurance creates.

Moving average. The unweighted mean of the previous n data points.

Nash equilibrium. A situation in which none of the participants want to change strategies, given what the others are doing.

Network externality. The effect each additional user of a product or service has on the value of that product or service to existing users.

Noncooperative game. A game in which the players cannot negotiate binding contracts.

Nonexcludable consumption. Nonpreventable consumption by someone who did not pay for a good or service.

Non-rival consumption. Consumption by one person that does not prevent simultaneous consumption by another person.

Normal rate of return. A profit rate that is high enough to retain current factors of production in an industry or occupation and low enough not to attract new entrants. (The normal rate of return will equal the opportunity cost of the factors.)

Normative economics. Using values to identify the best options.

Objective probability. An estimate of probability based on observed frequencies.

Oligopolist. A firm with only a few rivals or a firm with only a few large rivals.

Opportunism. Taking advantage of a situation without regard for the interests of others.

Opportunity cost. The value of a resource in its next best use. (The opportunity cost of a product consists of the other goods and services we cannot have because we have chosen to produce the product in question.)

Out-of-pocket price. The amount of money a consumer herself pays for a good or service.

Output. The good or service that emerges from a production process.

Pareto optimal. An allocation of resources is Pareto optimal if no reallocation of resources is possible that will improve the well being of one person without worsening the well being of another.

Percentage adjustment. Percentage adjustment of the past n periods of historic demand. (The adjustment is essentially a best guess of what is expected to happen in the next year.)

Point of service (POS) plan. Plan that allows members to see any physician but increases cost sharing for physicians outside the plan's network. (This arrangement has become so common that POS plans may not be labeled as such.)

Positive economics. Using objective analysis and evidence to answer questions about individuals, organizations, and societies.

Preemption. Building enough excess capacity in a market to discourage potential entrants.

Preferred provider organization (PPO). An insurance plan that contracts with a network of providers. (Network providers may be chosen for a variety of reasons, but a willingness to discount fees is usually required.)

Price discrimination. Selling similar products to different individuals at different prices.

Price elasticity of demand. The percentage change in sales volume associated with a 1 percent change in a product's price.

Principal. The organization or individual represented by an agent.

Prisoner's dilemma. A game in which the outcome both parties prefer is not an equilibrium.

Production to order. Setting prices and then filling customers' orders.

Production to stock. Producing output and then adjusting prices to sell what has been produced.

Profits. Total revenue minus total cost.

Public good. A good whose consumption is non-rival and nonexcludable.

Quantity demanded. The amount of a good or service that will be purchased at a specific price when all other factors are held constant.

Range. The difference between the largest and smallest values of a variable.

Rational decision-making. Choosing the course of action that gives you the best outcomes, given the constraints you face.

Return on assets. Profits divided by assets.

Return on equity. Profits divided by shareholder equity.

Risk aversion. The reluctance of a decision maker to accept an outcome with an uncertain payoff rather than a smaller, more certain outcome. (A risk-averse person would prefer getting $5 for sure to a gamble with a 50 percent chance of getting nothing and a 50 percent chance of getting $10.)

Risk neutrality. The indifference of a decision maker to risk. (A risk-neutral person would think that getting $5 for sure is as good as a gamble with a 50 percent chance of getting nothing and a 50 percent chance of getting $10.)

Risk seeking. The preference of a decision maker for risk. (A risk-seeking person would prefer a gamble with a 50 percent chance of getting nothing and a 50 percent chance of getting $10 to getting $5 for sure.)

Scarce resources. Anything useful in consumption or production that has alternative uses.

Seasonalized regression analysis. A least squares regression that includes variables that identify sub-periods (e.g., weeks) that historically have had above- or below-trend sales.

Sensitivity analysis. The process of varying the assumptions in an analysis over a reasonable range and observing how the outcome changes.

Shift in demand. A shift that occurs when a factor other than price of the product itself (e.g., consumer incomes) changes.

Shortage. Situation in which the quantity demanded at the prevailing price exceeds the quantity supplied.

Signaling. Sending messages that reveal information another party does not observe.

Societal perspective. A perspective that takes account of all costs and benefits, no matter to whom they accrue.

Staff model HMO. HMO that directly employs staff physicians to provide services.

Standard deviation. The square root of a variance.

Subjective probability. An individual's judgment about how likely a particular event is to occur.

Substitute. A product used instead of another product.

Sunk costs. Costs that have been incurred and cannot be recouped.

Supply curve. Curve that describes how much producers are willing to sell at different prices.

Supply shift. Shift that occurs when a factor (e.g., an input price) other than price of the product changes.

Tragedy of the commons. Over- or underuse of a resource that occurs when ownership of the resource is unclear and users produce externalities.

Underwriting. The process of assessing the risks associated with an insurance policy and setting the premium accordingly.

Utilization review. Analysis of patterns of resource use.

Variance. The expected squared deviation of a random variable from its expected value (If a variable takes the value 3 with a probability of 0.2, the value 6 with a probability of 0.3, and the value 9 with a probability of 0.5, its expected value is 6.9. Its variance is 5.49, which is $0.2 \times [3 - 6.9]^2 + 0.3 \times [6 - 6.9]^2 + 0.5 \times [9 - 6.9]^2$.)

Zero-sum game. A game in which any gains by one player must be matched by losses by another player.

INDEX

ABOUT THE AUTHOR

Robert H. Lee, PhD, is an associate professor in the Department of Health Policy and Management of the School of Medicine of the University of Kansas. Previously he worked at the University of North Carolina, the Health Policy Program of the Urban Institute, and the Brookings Institution. He has published more than 30 healthcare economics articles.